Osteosarcoma – Diagnosis, Mechanisms, and Translational Developments

Edited by Matthew Gregory Cable and Robert Lawrence Randall

Published in London, United Kingdom

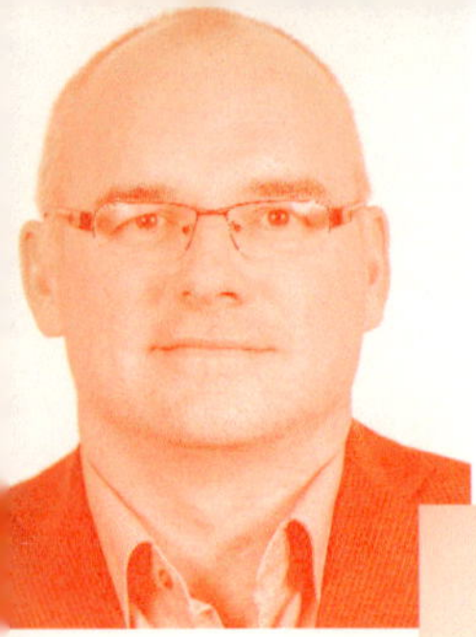
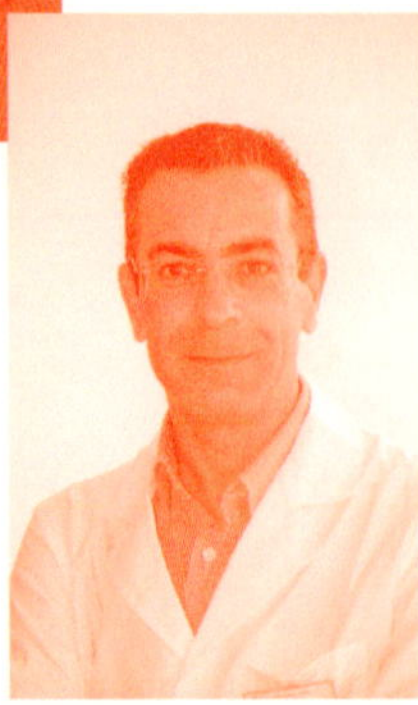
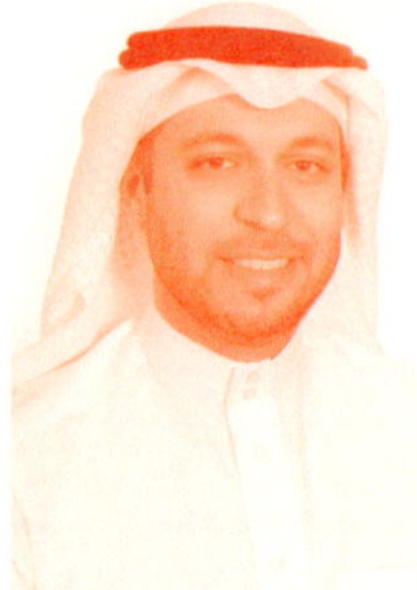
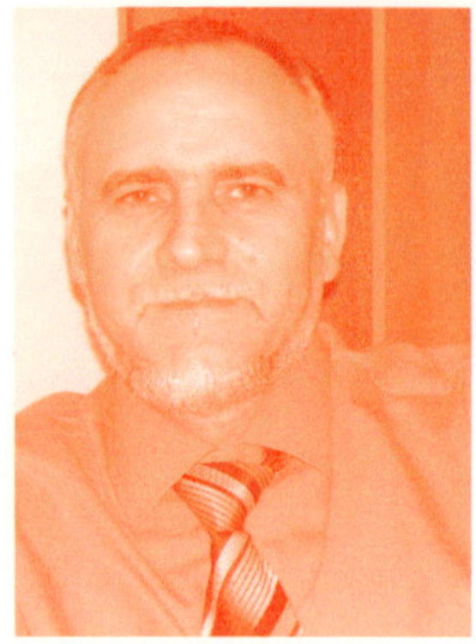
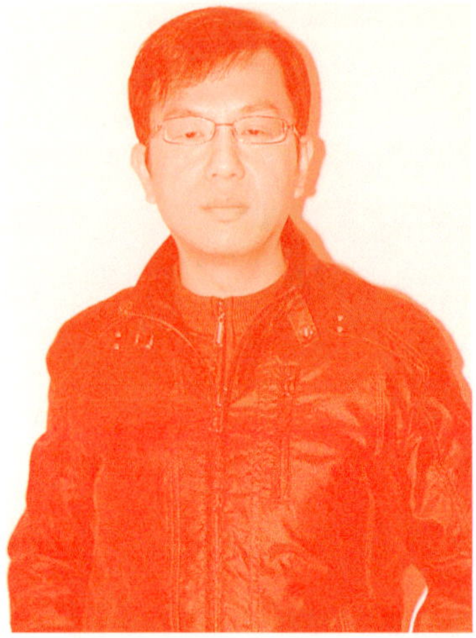
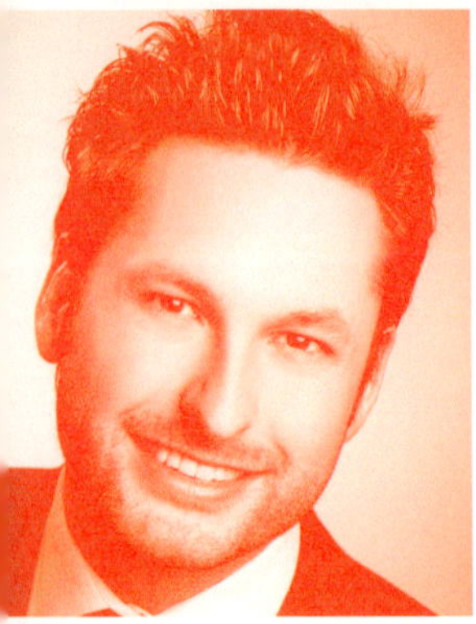
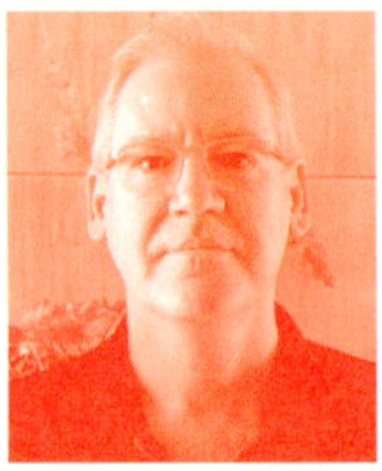

IntechOpen

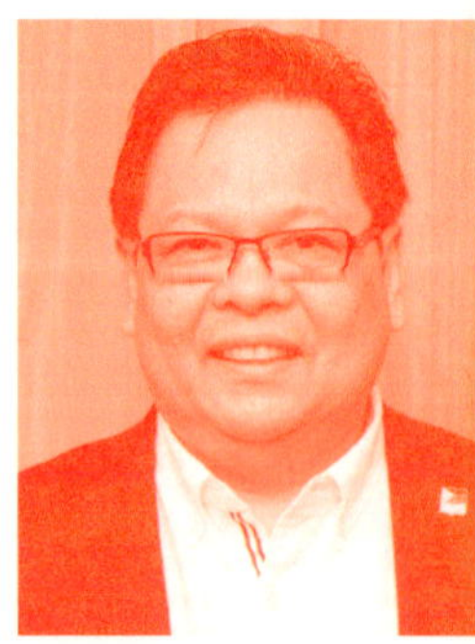
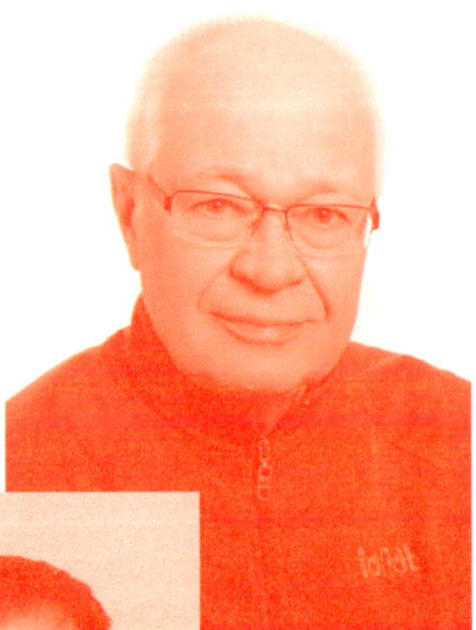
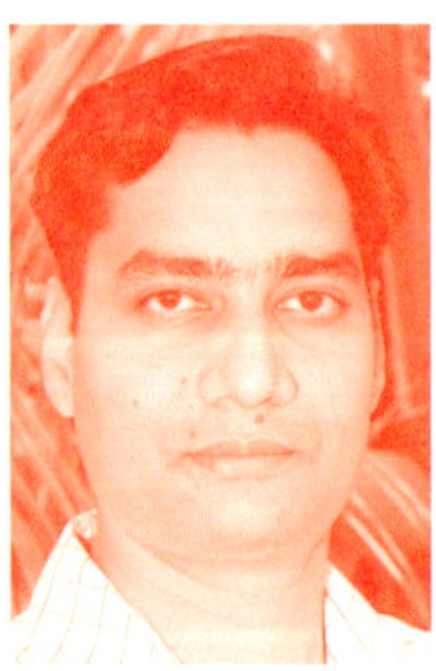
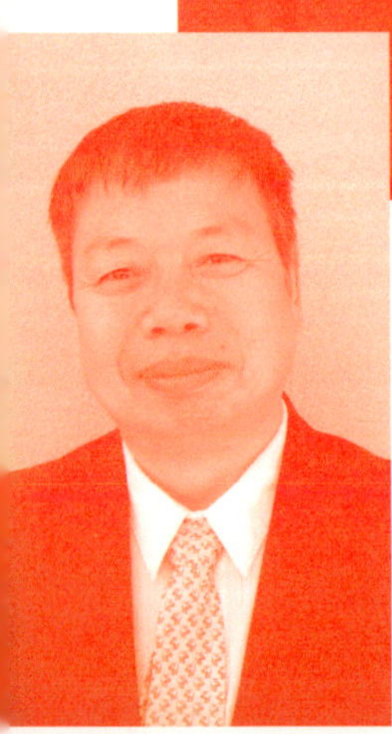
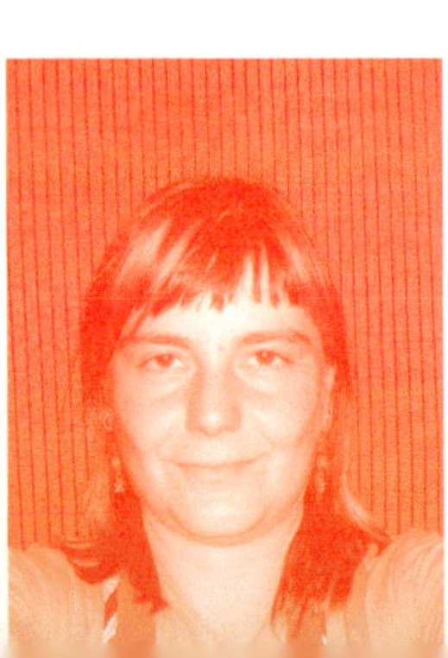
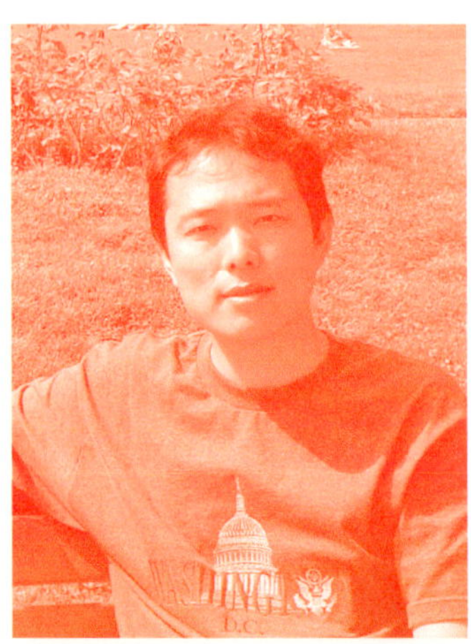

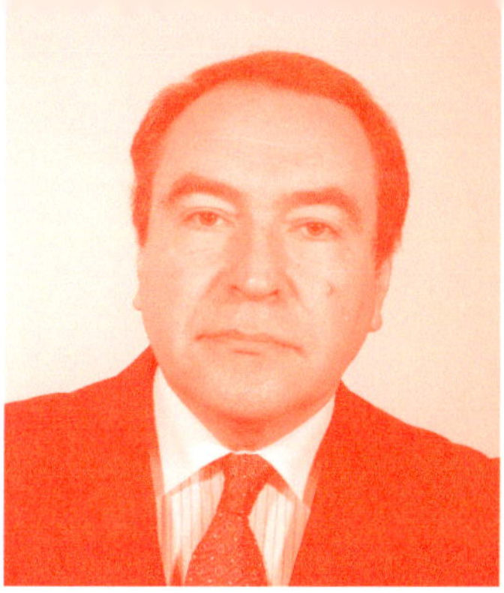
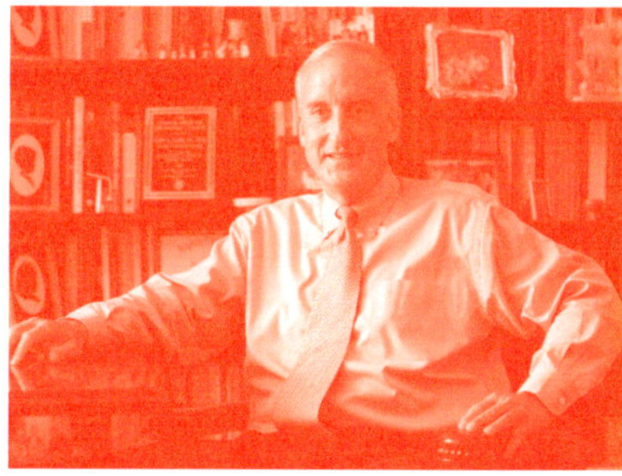
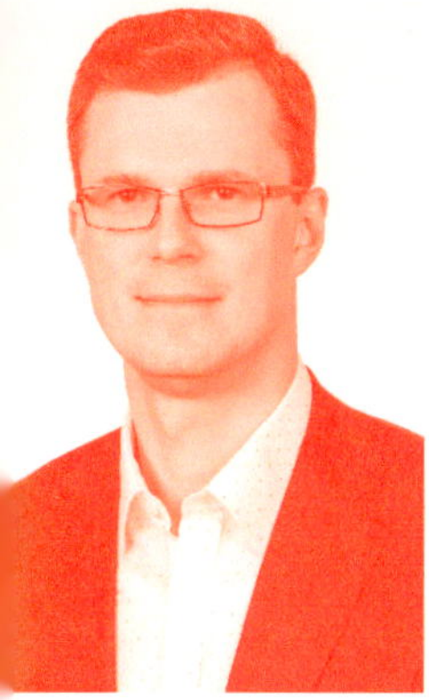
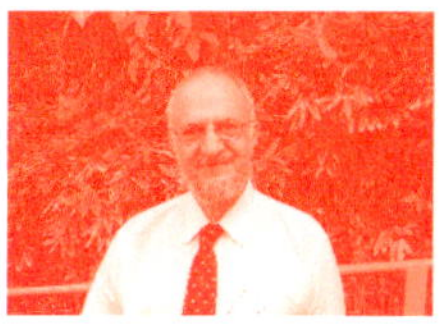
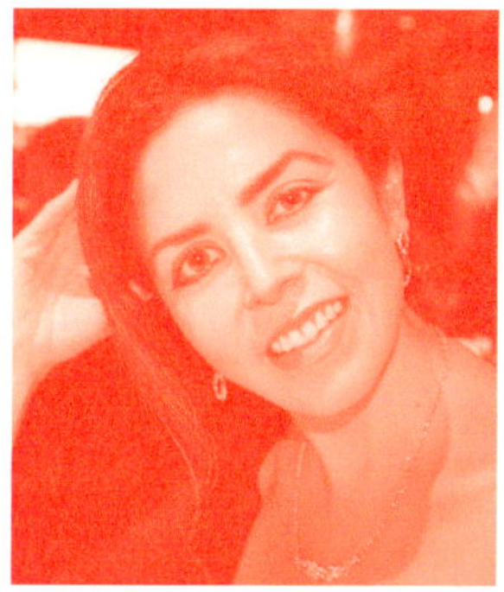

Supporting open minds since 2005

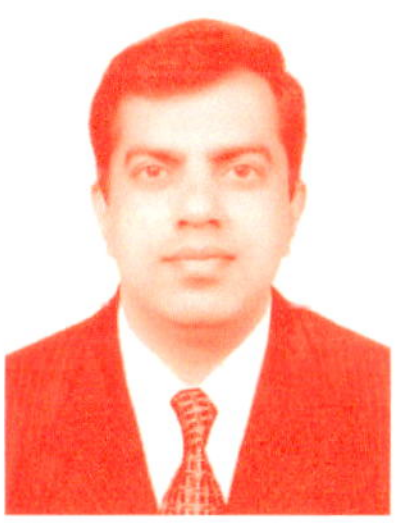
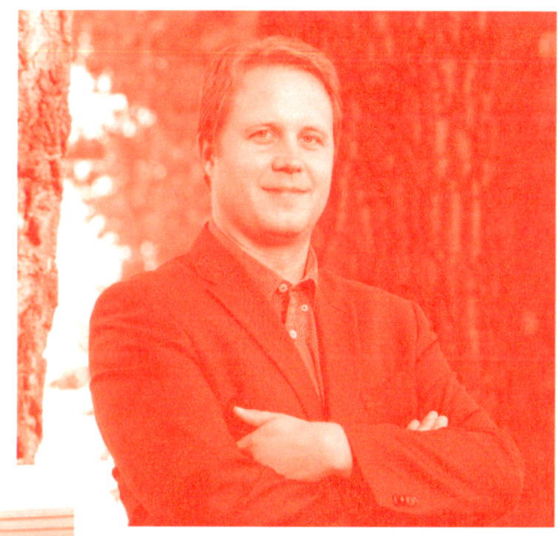
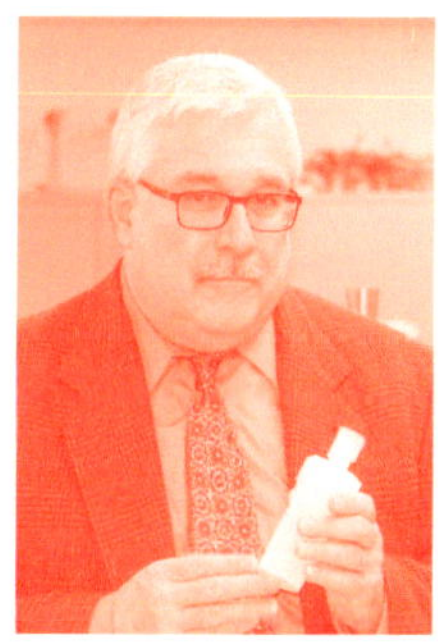
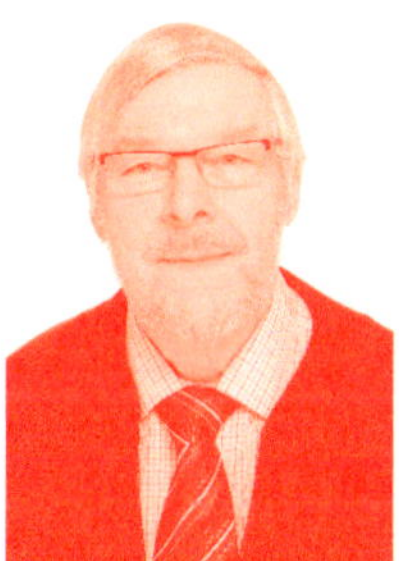
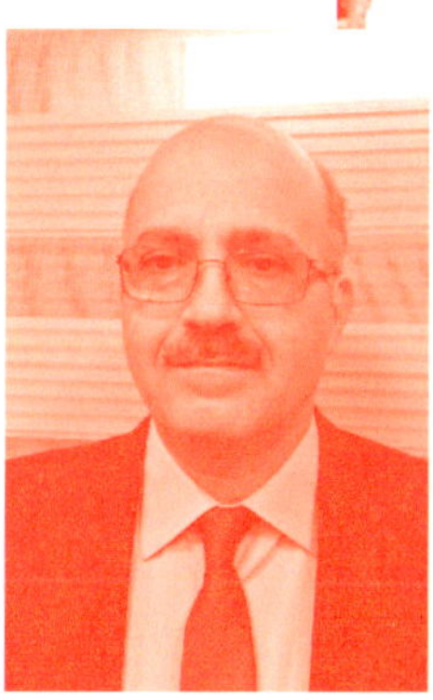
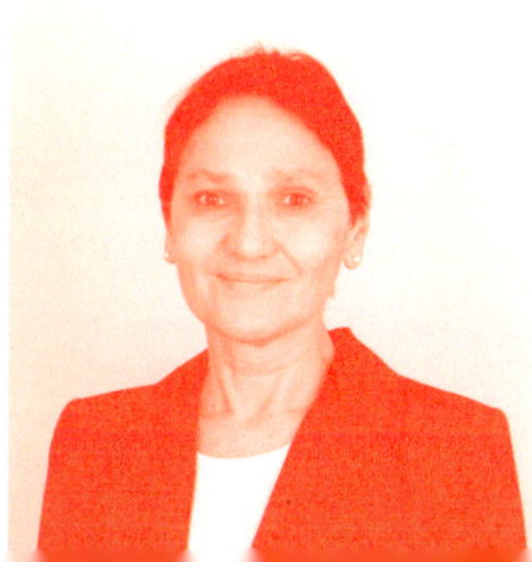
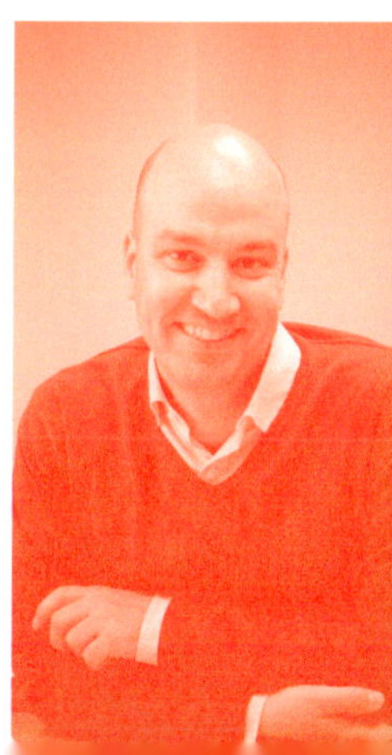

Osteosarcoma - Diagnosis, Mechanisms, and Translational Developments
http://dx.doi.org/10.5772/intechopen.73987
Edited by Matthew Gregory Cable and Robert Lawrence Randall

Contributors
Mulazim Hussain Bukhari, Farwa Batool, Samina Qamar, Mandeep Bedi, Kanya Honoki, Shingo Kishi, Yasuhito Tanaka, Hiroki Kuniyasu, Christos Valavanis, Gabriela Stanc, Maxim Rykov, Elmira Sengapova, Matthew Gregory Cable, Scott Barnett

First published in London, United Kingdom, 2019 by IntechOpen
IntechOpen is the global imprint of INTECHOPEN LIMITED, registered in England and Wales, registration number: 11086078, 7th floor, 10 Lower Thames Street, London, EC3R 6AF, United Kingdom
Printed in Croatia

British Library Cataloguing-in-Publication Data
A catalogue record for this book is available from the British Library

Additional hard and PDF copies can be obtained from orders@intechopen.com

Osteosarcoma - Diagnosis, Mechanisms, and Translational Developments
Edited by Matthew Gregory Cable and Robert Lawrence Randall
p. cm.
Print ISBN 978-1-83968-014-4
Online ISBN 978-1-83968-015-1
eBook (PDF) ISBN 978-1-83968-016-8

For EU product safety concerns:
IN TECH d.o.o., Prolaz Marije Krucifikse Kozulić 3, 51000 Rijeka, Croatia, info@intechopen.com or visit our website at intechopen.com.

Meet the editors

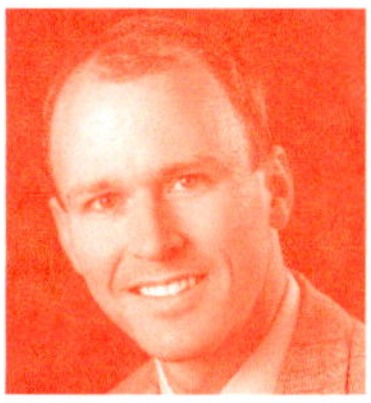

Dr. Matthew G. Cable is an assistant professor in the Louisiana State University Health Science Center Department of Orthopaedic Surgery, Division of Musculoskeletal Oncology. Dr. Cable completed medical training at the University of Chicago Pritzker School of Medicine, orthopedic surgery residency at the Detroit Medical Center/Wayne State University, and a two-year Sarcoma Advanced Clinical and Research fellowship at the Huntsman Cancer Institute and Primary Children's Hospital at the University of Utah. He is a member of the Musculoskeletal Tumor Society and the Connective Tissue Oncology Society. He is an orthopedic oncologist specializing in the surgical treatment of adult and pediatric tumors, including osteosarcoma, and has numerous publications and book chapters pertaining to musculoskeletal oncology.

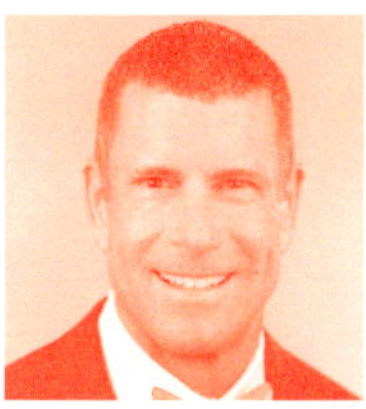

Robert Lawrence Randall, MD, FACS, is the chair of the Department of Orthopaedic Surgery at the University of California, Davis in Sacramento. Dr. Randall's clinical practice and research focus on musculoskeletal surgical oncology and on building leading-edge transdisciplinary teams to combat rare cancers of connective tissue in children and adults. His translational research efforts have been recognized internationally, including his work as chief of the Sarcoma Array Research Consortium (SARC) lab, a laboratory investigating the molecular genetic mechanisms that give rise to sarcomas; his development of a genetically engineered mouse model at the University of Utah (in cooperation with Nobel Prize cowinner Mario Capecchi); and his technical advancements in limb salvage surgery.
Dr. Randall is a professor of Orthopaedic Surgery and holds the David Linn Chair in Orthopaedic Surgery.

Contents

Preface XI

Section 1
Introduction 1

Chapter 1 3
Introductory Chapter: Integrating Basic Science with a Multidisciplinary Clinical Approach for Osteosarcoma
by Scott Barnett and Matthew G. Cable

Section 2
Osteosarcoma Diagnosis and Characterization 9

Chapter 2 11
Differential Diagnosis of Osteogenic Tumors in the Context of Osteosarcoma
by Mulazim Hussain Bukhari, Samina Qamar and Farwa Batool

Section 3
Basic Science and Translational Treatments 37

Chapter 3 39
Long Noncoding RNAs in Osteosarcoma: Mechanisms and Potential Clinical Implications
by Christos Valavanis and Gabriela Stanc

Chapter 4 81
A Novel Strategy of Dual Inhibition of Distinct Metabolic Features in Osteosarcoma
by Shingo Kishi, Kanya Honoki, Yasuhito Tanaka and Hiroki Kuniyasu

Chapter 5 97
Treatment of Children with Osteosarcoma
by Maxim Yu. Rykov and Elmira R. Sengapova

Preface

The predecessor to this edition was titled *Osteosarcoma: Biology, Behavior, and Mechanisms*, and was the brainchild of my good friend Dr. Kurt Weiss and colleague Dr. Kanya Honoki. They sought to draw attention and enthusiasm to the recent advances in basic and clinical science research pertaining to osteosarcoma. There had been a relative stagnation in clinical advances over past decades in this rare cancer in comparison to other oncologic diseases. We began to understand the molecular biology and genetics of osteosarcoma but were unable to translate this into longer survival or improved prognosis. However, this was on the precipice of change with recent technological developments in big data genomics, improved understanding of molecular pathways, and discovery of new methods of epigenetic tumor regulation.

This edition is titled *Osteosarcoma—Diagnosis, Mechanisms, and Translational Developments*, and focuses on recent advancements and novel ideas in osteosarcoma research. In a manner of speaking, we have taken the multidisciplinary mindset essential for treating osteosarcoma and broadened it to include other areas of cancer research. By learning from gains in other areas of oncology, such as new lncRNAs, the understanding of cancer metabolism and oxidative phosphorylation, and new chemotherapy agents, we can apply them to the niche of osteosarcoma for treatment development. By drawing more attention to these novel and clever discoveries, we hope to continue this enthusiasm for advancements in basic and translational research in the field of osteosarcoma.

Matthew Gregory Cable, MD
Assistant Professor,
Louisiana State University Health Sciences Center,
Department of Orthopaedic Surgery,
Division of Musculoskeletal Oncology,
New Orleans, USA

Robert Lawrence Randall
University of California,
USA

Section 1

Introduction

Chapter 1

Introductory Chapter: Integrating Basic Science with a Multidisciplinary Clinical Approach for Osteosarcoma

Scott Barnett and Matthew G. Cable

1. Introduction

Primary bone neoplasms are relatively uncommon. Among these tumors, osteosarcoma is the most common bone sarcoma, comprising approximately 35% of all malignant bone tumors [1]. Osteosarcoma affects approximately 500 children and adolescents annually in the United States with incidence peaking in the second decade of life during periods of rapid bone turnover and growth spurts [2]. Osteosarcoma arises from sites of rapid bone turnover, making the distal femur, proximal tibia and proximal humerus the most typical locations [3].

Although a genetic predisposition with mutations in various tumor-suppressor genes incurs a higher likelihood of developing osteosarcoma, most cases of osteosarcoma are sporadic. These chromosomal abnormalities yield defects in proteins involved in cell cycle regulation, resulting in uncontrolled cell proliferation [4]. These mutations are seen in a variety of disorders including Li-Fraumeni syndrome, which involves the p53 gene, or retinoblastoma, which involves the RB1 gene [5]. Some existing bone diseases such as Paget disease, fibrous dysplasia, enchondromatosis, and hereditary multiple exostosis in addition to environmental risk factors, including radiation, have been identified as contributors to developing osteosarcoma.

Osteosarcoma serves as a broad term used to envelop the several different types of osteosarcoma that exist. These subtypes distinguish themselves through both clinical appearance as well as behavior. Unfortunately, the histological pictures of bone tumors do not definitively differentiate between osteogenic sarcoma, benign tumors, or other malignancies of bone [6]. Therefore, incorporation of both radiological and clinical tools is required to make the final diagnosis of osteogenic sarcoma [7].

In the setting of osteosarcoma, advanced imaging is warranted to evaluate the extent of tumor invasion, neurovascular involvement, bone marrow replacement, and presence of discontinuous metastases. Combination of MRI and CT imaging are helpful in demonstrating both soft tissue parameters of the tumor as well as cortical integrity and the presence of pathologic fracture [8, 9]. New focus on advanced techniques in medical image processing for the detection and analysis of osteosarcoma aims to better evaluate tumor locations, size, infiltrations of surrounding tissues, and identify the presence of satellite metastasis. Current research work utilizes positron emission tomography (PET) combined with MRI volumetry to better assess histological responses in bone sarcoma afflicted individuals, yielding

IntechOpen

improvements in classification accuracy compared single modality evaluation [10]. The coupling of FDG-PET and MRI volumes offers improved prognostic and predicting capabilities for assessing the aggressiveness of tumors and aiding earlier clinical decisions regarding the utility of treatment options for patients.

A multidisciplinary approach is used for the treatment of patients with osteosarcoma, offering survival rates of greater than 70% with metastatic disease [11, 12]. For high-grade osteosarcoma, treatment involves preoperative chemotherapy, wide surgical resection, and postoperative chemotherapy. Intratumor heterogeneity, a resultant of tumor evolution, is the fundamental challenge in cancer medicine. From heterogeneity stems disease relapse, metastatic behaviors, and drug resistance [13]. Recent studies of cancer stem cells report a metabolism pathway that is predominantly through oxidative phosphorylation rather than glycolysis [14]. Targeting this metabolic pathway presents a potential therapeutic option against tumor cells. Within the mitochondria, a "two metabolic hit" theory has been proposed to utilize the synergistic effects of combining oxidative phosphorylation inhibition with c-Myc inhibition, which target both the oxidative phosphorylation-dominant cancer stem cells and glycolysis-dominant non-cancer stem cells [15]. Novel compounds such as pterostilbene and honokiol have emerged as dual metabolic inhibition compounds that may lead to improvements in osteosarcoma prognosis, especially in the setting of metastatic disease [16].

Additional studies have shown that molecules belonging to the non-protein coding transcriptome may play essential roles in biological processes [17]. These non-protein coding RNAs are involved in gene expression regulation and have been found to play an important role in cancer development, progression, and chemoresistance of different tumors, including osteosarcoma [18]. Non-coding RNAs have emerged as potential prognostic biomarkers and therapeutic targets, being involved in cell signal transduction pathways, cell cycle and death regulation, chromatin remodeling, and gene expression regulation at both transcriptional and posttranscriptional levels [19]. Several tumors, such as urothelial carcinoma, colon carcinoma, and hepatocellular carcinoma have exhibited aberrant expression of non-coding RNAs, suggesting a new means of observation that may be exploited for diagnostic, prognostic preventative, or therapeutic processes [20]. A large number of long non-coding chain RNAs (lncRNAs) with oncogenic or tumor suppressive activity are differentially expressed in osteosarcoma. MALAT-1 (metastasis-associated lung adenocarcinoma transcript 1), a lncRNA involved in recruiting mRNA splicing factors to transcription sites, is overexpressed in osteosarcoma and has expression levels linked to tumor metastatic potential [21]. The identification of lncRNAs serves as a catalyst for further research validating lncRNAs as prognostic and predictive biomarkers, therapeutic targets, and structural models for future mimicking pharmaceutical agents.

New targetable compounds generate hope for novel osteosarcoma treatment regimens, specifically with the affected pediatric population where chemotherapy has become the mainstay of treatment. Surgical resection yielded a high frequency of relapse and metastasis for children with osteosarcoma, shifting the focus to intense chemotherapy [22]. Similar to the discovery of lncRNAs, new molecular biologic factors that determine sensitivity to chemotherapy, invasive and metastatic potential of the tumor, and the prognosis of the disease have been elucidated in recent pediatric osteosarcoma research. Expression of methylguanine methyltransferase (MGMT) as well as MGMT methylation is correlated with poor histological response in osteosarcoma patients undergoing cisplatin treatment [23]. Other molecular factors such as vascular endothelial growth factor (VEGF) and c-Myc are under intense focus for characterizing tumor behavior, response to treatment, and dictating further treatment protocols [24]. Although there is significant relapse and

DOI: http://dx.doi.org/10.5772/intechopen.87992

refractory rates for children diagnosed with metastatic osteosarcoma, comprehensive assessments of these markers for histological response to chemotherapy may enhance current treatment protocols and guide future regimens.

Emphasis on basic science research remains a prime avenue for uncovering molecular mechanisms and biologic pathways that may lead to additional targeted therapies, less-toxic agents, and improved long-term survival in osteosarcoma [25]. Molecular biomarkers such as non-coding RNAs and cell-cycle regulator proteins are an area of current interest for the development of sensitive screening modalities as well as target-selective chemotherapeutic drugs. Progress in combined advanced imaging techniques offer better, non-invasive means for evaluating tumor, size, location and behavior, which facilitates clinical decision making. Treatment of osteosarcoma, an aggressive and malignant tumor, requires a multidisciplinary approach that incorporates progressive basic science research at all levels of care including diagnosis, treatment, and surveillance.

Acknowledgements

We thank the international colleagues and contributors in this book for helping to better understand osteosarcoma and the other often-overlooked rare diseases that affect our patients and their families. We also are grateful for Ms. Martina Usljebrka and Sara Petanjek for their assistance in editing and bringing this text to fruition.

Author details

Scott Barnett and Matthew G. Cable*
Department of Orthopaedic Surgery, Louisiana State University Health Sciences Center, New Orleans, Louisiana, USA

*Address all correspondence to: mcabl1@lsuhsc.edu

References

[1] Dorfman H, Vanel D, Czerniak B, Park Y, Kotz R, Unni K. Introduction, WHO Classification of Tumours of Soft Tissue and Bone. In: Fletcher C, editor. 4th ed. IARC; 2013

[2] Horner MJ, Ries LAG, Krapcho M, et al. SEER Cancer Statistics 1975-2016. Bethesda, MD: National Cancer Institute. Available at: http://seer.cancer.gov/csr/1975_2016. Accessed [6 July 2019]

[3] Bielack SS, Kempf-Bielack B, Delling G, et al. Prognostic factors in high-grade osteosarcoma of the extremities or trunk: An analysis of 1.702 patients treated on neoadjuvant cooperative osteosarcoma study group protocols. Journal of Clinical Oncology. 2002;**20**:776-790

[4] Hayden JB, Hoang BH. Osteosarcoma: Basic science and clinical implications. The Orthopedic Clinics of North America. 2006;**37**:1-7

[5] Wang LL. Biology of osteogenic sarcoma. Cancer Journal. 2005;**11**:294-305

[6] Klein MJ, Siegal GP. Osteosarcoma: Anatomic and histologic variants. American Journal of Clinical Pathology. 2006;**125**:55-581

[7] Murphy MD. World Health Organization classification of bone and soft tissue tumors: Modifications and implications for radiologists. Seminars in Musculoskeletal Radiology. 2007;**11**(3):201-214

[8] Scully SP, Ghert MA, Zurakowski D, Thompson RC, Gebhardt MC. Pathologic fracture in osteosarcoma: Prognostic importance and treatment implications. The Journal of Bone and Joint Surgery. American Volume. 2002;**84**:49-57

[9] Bedi SS, Agarwal J, Agarwal P. Image fusion techniques and quality assessment parameters for clinical diagnosis: A review. International Journal of Advanced Research in Computer and Communication Engineering. 2013;**2**(2):1153-1157

[10] Eugene T, Corradini N, Carlier T, Dupas B, Leux C, Bodet-Milin C. 18F-FDG-PET/CT in initial staging and assessment of early response to chemotherapy of pediatric rhabdomyosarcomas. Nuclear Medicine Communications. 2012;**3**(10):1089-1095

[11] Meyers PA, Schwartz CI, Krailo M. Osteosarcoma: The addition of muramyl tripeptide to chemotherapy improves overall survival. Journal of Clinical Oncology. 2008;**26**:633-638

[12] Ferrari S, Smeland S, Mercuri M. Neoadjuvant chemotherapy with high-dose ifosfamide, high-dose methotrexate, cisplatin, and doxorubicin for patients with localized osteosarcoma of the extremity. Journal of Clinical Oncology. 2005;**23**:8845-8852

[13] Bonnet D, Dick JE. Human acute myeloid leukemia is organized as a hierarchy that originates form a primitive hematopoietic cell. Nature Medicine. 1997;**3**:730-737

[14] Vander Heiden MG, Cantley LC, Thompson CB. Understanding the Warburg effect: The metabolic requirements of cell proliferation. Science. 2009;**324**:1029-1033

[15] Lin CY, Loven J, Rahl PB, Paranal RM, Burge CB, Bradner JE. Transcriptional amplification in tumor cells with elevated c-Myc. Cell. 2012;**151**:56-67

[16] Hahm ER, Singh KB, Singh SV. C-Myc is a novel target of cell cycle arrest by honokiol in prostate cancer cells. Cell Cycle. 2016;**15**(17):2309-2320

[17] Sandberg K, Samson WK, Ji H. Decoding noncoding RNA: The long and short of it. Circulation Research. 2013;**113**(3):240-241

[18] Crea F, Clermont PI, Parolia A, Wang Y, Helgason CD. The non-coding transcriptome as a dynamic regulator of cancer metastasis. Cancer Metastasis Reviews. 2013;**33**(1):1-16

[19] Huarte M. The emerging role of lncRNAs in cancer. Nature Medicine. 2015;**21**(11):1253-1261

[20] Min L, Garbutt C, Tu C, Hornicek F, Duan Z. Potentials for long noncoding RNAs (kncRNAs) in sarcoma: From biomarkers to therapeutic targets. International Journal of Molecular Sciences. 2017;**18**(4):731

[21] Smolle MA, Pichler M. The role of long non-coding RNAs in osteosarcoma. Noncoding RNA. 2018;**4**(1):7

[22] Punanov YA, Andreeva TV, Gafton GI, et al. The results of combined therapy in children and adolescents with osteosarcoma. Oncopediatrics. 2014;**1**(2):49-53

[23] Cui Q, Li D, Liu C, et al. The significance of MGMT protein detection in evaluation of osteosarcoma necrosis rate after cisplatin chemotherapy. Bosnian Journal of Basic Medical Sciences. 2011;**11**(2):80-83

[24] Rossi B, Schinzari G, Maccauro G, et al. Neoadjuvant multidrug chemotherapy including high-dose methotrexate modifies VEGF expression in osteosarcoma: An immunohistochemical analysis. BMC Musculoskeletal Disorders. 2010;**11**(34):1471-2474

[25] Messerschmit PJ, Garcia RM, Abdul-Karim FW, Greenfield EM, Getty PJ. Osteosarcoma. The Journal of the American Academy of Orthopaedic Surgeons. 2009;**17**(8):515-527

Section 2

Osteosarcoma Diagnosis and Characterization

Chapter 2

Differential Diagnosis of Osteogenic Tumors in the Context of Osteosarcoma

Mulazim Hussain Bukhari, Samina Qamar and Farwa Batool

Abstract

Primary bone tumors are rare, but osteosarcoma (OS) is the fourth commonest non-hematological primary neoplasm of the bone in the adolescence, and the other three commonest neoplasms, in descending order, are leukemia, brain tumors, and lymphoma. The commonest presenting complaints are swelling and aches. These tumors cannot be diagnosed without the help of radiology. There is a wide age range of these neoplasms commonly appearing in the second and third decade of life with a peak incidence in early teens. Males are affected more than females. The exact cause of osteosarcoma is unknown. However, a number of risk factors, like genetic predisposition, some existing bone diseases, environmental risk factors, and radiations, have been identified. If the bone tumors are viewed by clinical, radiological, and histopathological perspectives, the correct diagnosis can be made easily. Chemotherapy combined with surgery is the standard treatment modality with better 5-year survival rates. Elevated AKP is an important prognostic factor in this malignancy.

Keywords: aggressive osteoblastoma, osteogenic tumors, osteoma, osteoid osteoma, osteoblastoma, osteogenic sarcoma

1. Introduction

Primary neoplasm of the bones is relatively uncommon. Among these tumors, the osteosarcoma is the commonest primary malignant tumor, comprising of approximately 35% of all bone malignant tumors, followed by others like chondrosarcoma (25%), Ewing sarcoma (EWS) (16%), and chordomas (8%). This malignant tumor can arise from any bone, mainly usually in the metaphyseal (growth plates) long bones of the extremities, but the jaw, pelvis, and ribs may be the sites of origin [1].

The nomenclature of bone tumors are described in "the World Health Organization (WHO)" classification system [2]. We are adopting a table from this classification to review the pathological diagnostic criteria of these lesions. A number of variants of osteosarcoma exist, including conventional types (osteoblastic, chondroblastic, fibroblastic, telangiectatic, multifocal, parosteal, and periosteal) (**Table 1**) [3].

The histological pictures of bone tumors alone are not enough to make a differentiation between osteosarcoma and benign tumors or other malignancies of the bone; therefore, radiological and clinical help is needed to make the final diagnosis of osteogenic sarcoma. Therefore, the chapter will not only address osteosarcoma but will also discuss all osteogenic tumors stepwise [1].

Benign	Intermediate	Malignant
Osteoma	Osteoblastoma	Low-grade central osteosarcoma (OS)
Osteoid osteoma		Conventional OS Chondroblastic OS Fibroblastic OS Osteoblastic OS
		Telangiectatic OS
		Small cell OS
		Parosteal OS
		Periosteal OS
		High-grade surface OS
		Secondary OS

Table 1.
WHO-based classification of osteogenic tumors of the bone.

This chapter will mainly focus on general clinical, imaging, and histopathological characteristics, which will aid in diagnosis but may add a little to advances in tumor biology or treatment of the multitude of bone tumors described in this chapter.

The exact cause of osteosarcoma is unknown. However, a number of risk factors, like genetic predisposition, some existing (Paget disease, fibrous dysplasia, enchondromatosis, and hereditary multiple exostoses and retinoblastoma) bone diseases, environmental risk factors, and radiations, have been identified.

Keeping in mind the importance of this malignancy, it is therefore important to understand the other osteogenic tumors before reaching the importance of osteosarcoma; we will describe the differential diagnosis of osteogenic tumors in the context of osteosarcoma.

2. Osteoma

It is a benign neoplasm exclusively seen in flat bone of skull and face. Microscopically it consists of the mature lamellar bone. Multiple osteomas are associated with Gardner's syndrome (colonic polyposis). Sometimes it involves other than the skull and face, as surface lesions of parosteal type (**Figure 1** and **Tables 1** and 2) [4].

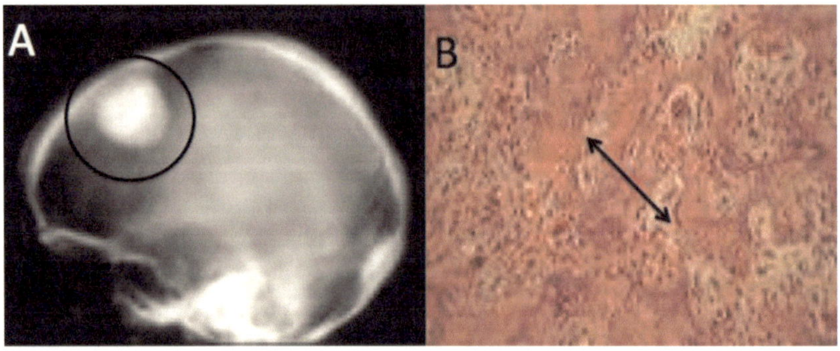

Figure 1.
Radiological aspect of osteoma, (A) shows sharply radiodense lesions (black ring), (B) photomicrograph (H&E 40x) similar to normal cortex, revealing mature bone (arrow), with less stroma and no atypia.

Features	Osteoma	Osteoid osteoma	Ossifying fibroma	Parosteal osteosarcoma
Site and location	Cortex of metaphysis (skull, facial bone)	Metaphysis	Metaphysis of the same bones	Metaphysis of long bone
Age in years	40–60 more in males	10–20 more in males	1–70 (wide range), and more in females	30–60 year (older age)
Clinical symptoms	No pain	With pain	No pain	Pain
Radiology	Well-circumscribed radiodense and without destructive features	A single <1.5 cm nidus that may be radiolucent or ossified and surrounded by a reactive bone	Well-demarcated radiolucent in the early stages and then progressive calcification	Continuity with the medullary component of the parent bone is not present. Appears to be attached to the surface of the parent none
Histology	Nodular or dome-shaped, dense cortical bone Consists of dense lamellar bone with or without Haversian canals and usually without a medullary component Medullary component consists of hematopoietic or fibroadipose tissue Regular large ossicles of mature bone	Lamellar bone with prominent osteoblastic rimming Osteoma may have focal areas of reactive bone with similar features but not cellular as compard to OO, see also (**Table 3**)	The stroma is fibrous and more cellular Small ossicles and irregular bony trabeculae, much less mature bone Psammoma bodies	Tumor osteoid is arranged in parallel arrays and separated by a bland fibroblastic stroma. With minimal atypia. Cartilage may be seen. Genetically, amplification of $12q^{13\text{-}15}$ seen with CDK4 and MDM2 genes. See also (**Table 9**) No other benign lesions seen (See **Table 9**)

Table 2.
Differential diagnosis of osteoma with osteoid osteoma, ossifying fibroma, and parosteal osteosarcoma.

3. Osteoid osteoma

It is a benign tumor of medullary metaphysis origin with a <2 cm lucent nidus, encompassed by the solid periosteal reaction. The characteristic features are its association with nocturnal pain (due to release of prostaglandin via Cox-1 and Cox-2 pathway) which can be relieved by aspirin, a salicylate analgesic. Histologically it comprised of three zones, nidus, fibrovascular stroma, and mineralized sclerotic bone. The nidus is composed of interconnected newly formed blood vessels and new bone-forming cells (osteoblasts and osteoid) [5–7] (**Table 3**, **Figure 2**). These tumors should be differentiated from osteomyelitis, stress fractures, osteoblastoma, osteosarcoma, and other lesions [8, 9].

4. Osteoblastoma

It arises from the medullary metaphysis, but most cases arise from spongiosa of the bone. It is a rare benign tumor of the bone. These tumors are now considered in intermediated groups as they may be locally aggressive and tend to affect the axial skeleton more often than osteoid osteoma. They are less painful and have poor response with aspirin [10, 11]. These have many osteoclasts like giant cells and less

Features	Osteoid osteoma	Osteomyelitis	Stress fracture	Osteoblastoma	Ossifying fibroma	Osteosarcoma
Site and location	Cortex of metaphysis	Not site specific	Not site specific	Medulla of metaphysis	Same bones	Metaphysis of long bone
Age in years	5–30 More in males	Any age	Old age	Mean age 20 (10–73) More in females	Wide range (1–70)	Older age
Clinical symptoms	Severe pain	Pain, fever	Pain	Not severe pain	No pain	Pain
Radiology	A single <1.5 cm nidus that may be radiolucent or ossified and surrounded by a reactive bone	Bone scan demonstrates central area of reduced uptake representing an avascular area of purulent material	Positive findings include sclerosis, periosteal reaction/elevation, cortical thickening, and a fracture line	Well-circumscribed nondestructive but sometimes with secondary ABC changes Some have central nidus >2 cm The lesions are predominantly lytic, with a rim of reactive sclerosis	Well-demarcated radiolucent in the early stages and then progressive calcification	Continuity with the medullary component of the parent bone is not present. Appears to be attached to the surface of the parent none MRI and CT are more helpful
Histology	Irregular trabeculae of lamellar bone with prominent osteoblastic rimming Loose fibrovascular stroma See also (**Table 2**)	No central nidus Presence of neutrophils, lymphocytes, macrophages, etc. (acute or chronic inflammatory cell infiltrate)	Zonal pattern with central, more mature, denser bone and peripheral woven bone Cartilage with endochondral ossification may be present	Irregular anastomosing trabeculae of osteoid and woven bone Variable mineralization and thickness of woven osteoid trabeculae. No central maturation like nudus Intralesional hemorrhages like ABC and numerous osteoclast-like giant cells No peripheral rim of fibrovascular tissue like in nidus Epithelioid aggressive variant with large atypical epithelioid like osteoblasts may confuse with OS, but take guidance from radiology. See (**Tables 2** and **4**)	The stroma is fibrous and more cellular Small ossicles and irregular bone Trabeculae, much less mature bone Psammoma bodies	Tumor osteoid is arranged in parallel arrays and separated by a hypocellular fibroblastic stroma The spindle cells between bony trabeculae instead of fat and hematopoietic tissue as seen in OS Lacks the fibrovascular stroma and osteoblastic rimming of osteoid osteoma May show cartilage component. See (**Tables 4–8**) for IHC

Table 3.
Differential diagnosis of osteoid osteoma with osteomyelitis, stress fracture, osteoblastoma, ossifying fibroma, and osteosarcoma.

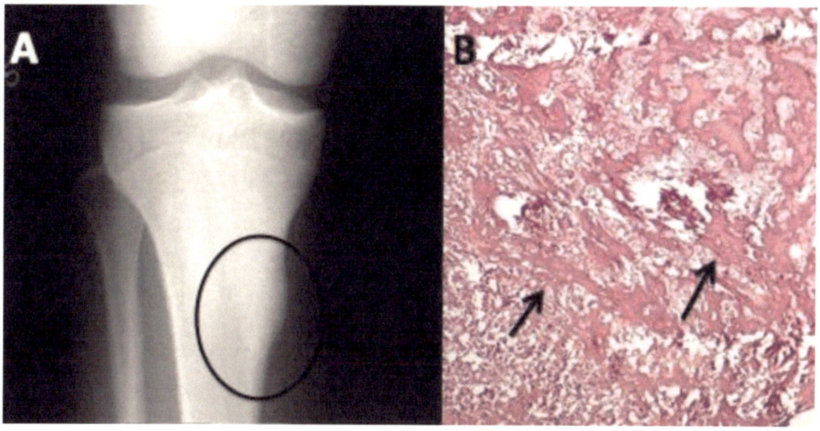

Figure 2.
Radiology of the osteoid osteoma (A) shows sharply radiodense lesions with nidus (black ring), similar to normal cortex, (B) photomicrograph (40X) of osteoid osteomas reveals irregular trabeculae of lamellar bone with prominent osteoblastic rimming and loose fibrovascular stroma (arrows).

Features	Osteoblastoma	Osteoid osteoma	Osteosarcoma	Giant cell tumors	Aneurysmal bone cyst (ABC)
Site and location	Medulla of metaphysis	Cortex of metaphysis	Metaphysis	Metaphysis of epiphysis	Diaphysis
Age in years	Mean age 20 (10–70) More in females	5–30 More in males	10–25	>20 Up to 40	Younger 10–20
Clinical symptoms	Not severe pain	Severe pain	Pain	No pain	No pain
Radiology	Well-circumscribed nondestructive but sometimes with ABC changes Some have central nidus >2 cm. The lesions are predominantly lytic, with a rim of reactive sclerosis	A single < 1.5 cm nidus that may be radiolucent or ossified and surrounded by a reactive bone	Radiographically, osteosarcoma is poorly circumscribed with cortical destruction and evidence of periosteal reactive bone Permeative pattern of growth at the periphery	Soap bubble appearance	Lytic but demarcated Both processes may have similar presentations and radiographic findings and tend to involve the vertebra
Histology	Irregular anastomosing trabeculae of osteoid and woven bone Variable mineralization and thickness of woven osteoid trabeculae. No central maturation like nidus Intralesional hemorrhages like ABC and numerous osteoclast-like giant cells No peripheral rim of fibrovascular tissue like in nidus	Irregular trabeculae of lamellar bone with prominent osteoblastic rimming Loose fibrovascular stroma	Tumor osteoid is arranged in parallel arrays and separated by a hypocellular fibroblastic stroma. Atypia is common The spindle cells between bony trabeculae instead of fat and hematopoietic tissue as seen in OS Lacks the fibrovascular stroma and osteoblastic rimming of osteoid osteoma May show cartilage component	Sheets of giant cells and more in number and contain more nuclei Giant cell tumors contain mononuclear stromal cells	Small foci of reactive osteoid may be present in aneurysmal bone cysts, which should not be confused with osteoblastoma

Table 4.
Differential diagnosis of osteoblastoma with osteoid osteoma, osteosarcoma, giant cell tumors, and ABC.

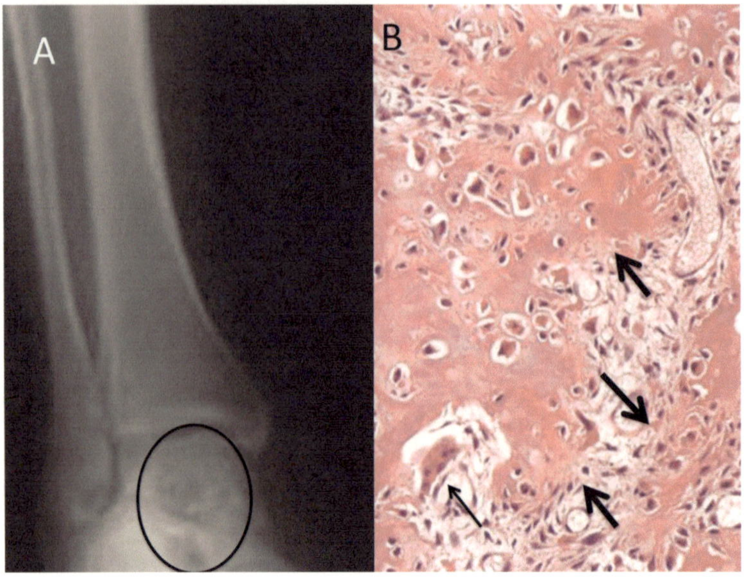

Figure 3.
(A) Radiology (left ankle bone) shows osteoblastoma, with well-circumscribed nondestructive but sometimes with ABC changes (ring). The lesions are predominantly lytic, with a rim of reactive sclerosis. (B) Photomicrograph (H&E 40X) showing irregular anastomosing trabeculae of osteoid and woven bone, variable mineralization, and thickness of woven osteoid trabeculae (thick arrows). Numerous osteoclast-like giant cells (thin arrow). No peripheral rim of fibrovascular tissue like in nidus.

rimming with osteoblasts, osteoid, and rich vascularity as compared to osteoid osteoma (**Table 4**, **Figure 3**) [6, 12, 13]. This is also called giant osteoid osteoma more than 2 cm in size; it does not have the surrounding reactive bone as compared to osteoid osteoma and is not associated with nocturnal aches [13].

4.1 Aggressive osteoblastoma

It is a rare variant of osteoblastoma, which commonly arises from the vertebrae, long bones, and bones of jaws; it is characterized by the presence of epithelioid osteoblasts in the stroma with aggressive behavior. The tumor has propensity for local invasion and recurrence, but still no metastasis has been seen in any case in the literature [14, 15].

5. Osteosarcoma (OS)

It is the most common primary bone tumors (20%) of mesenchymal origin second to multiple myeloma; the main histologic feature of this tumor is direct production of malignant osteoid from malignant cells without normal osteogenic process through fibrous and cartilage way; the cartilage or fibrous tissue may present elsewhere or in other osteogenic portions. Malignant osteoid is the characteristic finding of all types of OSs, and it is a eosinophilic, homogenous, glassy appearing lacelike material [16, 17].

Osteosarcoma is very rare in young children (0.5 cases per million per year in children <5 years). However, the incidence increases steadily with age [13].

It can affect all ages, but 75% appears in young age, it can affect all bones most commonly in metaphysis of long bones, and knee joint is commonly involved

(60%). There is no gender difference, but males are affected more as compared to females [13].

There are many morphological variants of OS with anastomosing, reticular osteoid and oval, spindled to epithelioid stromal cells. The cells may form rosettes to small sheets in different patterns. There are several subtypes of OS, which can be, differentiated on the basis of the site, degree of histological differentiation, and association with underlying disease [12, 13, 16, 17].

5.1 Conventional intermedullary OS

This type of OS shows the male predominance and bimodal age, pediatric and adult sarcoma. It has some association with hereditary effect, e.g., with mutation of RB gene, Li-Fraumeni syndrome, Ollier disease, fibrous dysplasia, and Paget disease (secondary OS). Radiation also plays a role in its pathogenesis. The long bones are commonly involved showing classical "Codman triangle" to moth-eaten picture due to permeation and destruction of medullary as well as cortical bone on radiology [18, 19].

It is composed of hyperchromatic cells forming sarcomatous component around the classical osteoid (**Figure 4**). This comprised of chondroblastic OS (25%), fibroblastic OS (25%), and osteoblastic OS (50%). Other subtypes are small cell-type OS, giant cell-rich OS, telengiactatic-type OS, surface-type OS, periosteal OS, and parosteal OS. Histologically it has two grades, low- and high-grade OS. Immunohistochemistry has some role in its differentiation from cartilage and other bone tumors, i.e., ALK, VIM, variable SMA, and desmin. The S100 is always negative except there is chondroid differentiation. EMA and keratin are negative in tumors [16, 20–23].

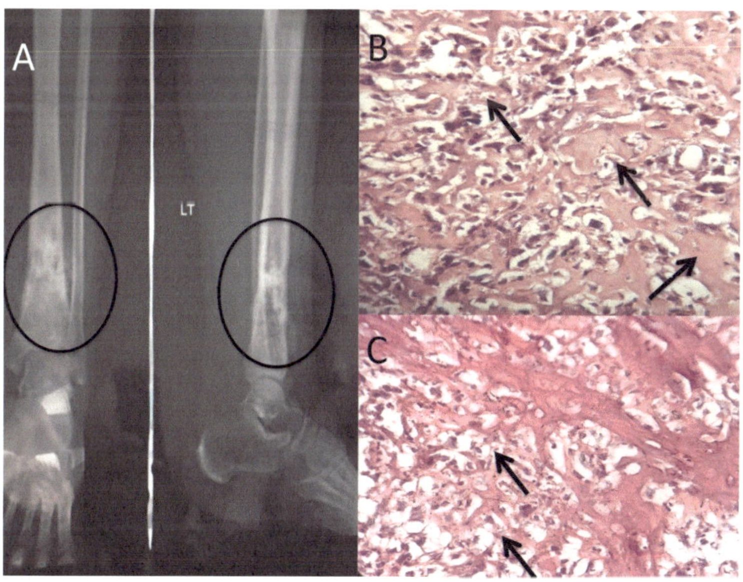

Figure 4.
Radiological examination (A) showing intramedullary OS of left lower tibia with osteolytic and sclerotic lesion in lower end above ankle joint (rings). There is a medullary and cortical destruction of bone. The photomicrograph of (B & C) (40X with H&E) based characteristic of conventional osteosarcoma, is the identification of osteoid (arrows), which is a dense, pink, amorphous extracellular material containing large amounts of collagen type I. (C) The tumor cells (atypical osteoblast) and cytoplasm are eosinophilic, are larger than normal osteoblasts (arrows), and vary in size with nuclear atypia.

6. Differential diagnosis of conventional OS

6.1 Fracture callus and stress fracture

Sometime fracture callus may be confused with OS, because there is formation of spindle cells and cartilage with new bones, but all these elements are arranged with orderly maturation as compared to haphazard and abrupt arrangement in OS (**Table 5**). Postmenopausal women may have insufficiency fractures in the pelvis resembling metastatic carcinoma [24, 25].

The osteoid and maturation level are the main difference between two lesions. The osteoid of the callus woven bone is mature and shows a parallel pattern with prominent osteoblastic rimming. Malignant osteoid is a eosinophilic, amorphous, fibrillary deposit between individual tumor cells or group of tumor cells. There are

Features	Conventional osteosarcoma (NOS)	Fracture callus	Ewing's sarcoma	Giant cell tumors (GCT)	Chondroblastoma
Site and location	Long bone	Not specific Can be of any site and any bone	Medulla of diaphysis and metaphysis	Metaphysis and epiphysis Rarely in vertebrae body	Epiphysis
Age in years	10–25	Any age	Children 4–20	>20 up to 40	Younger age 10–30
Clinical symptoms	Pain	May be pain		No pain	Pain
Radiology	Radiographically, osteosarcoma is poorly circumscribed with cortical destruction and evidence of periosteal reactive bone Permeative pattern of growth at the periphery	There may be increased translucency of the fracture during this stage, due to bone resorption	Metaphyseal or diaphyseal tumor with a predominantly lytic appearance. No bone matrix is radiographically identified Onion skin appearance in ES on radiology	Soap bubble appearance	Sharp and lytic lesions Fine calcification
Histology	Tumor osteoid is arranged in parallel arrays and separated by a hypocellular osteoblastic stroma. Atypia and mitosis are common The small cells between bony osteoid. CD99, LCA, CK, and S-100 are negative	There is spindle cell proliferation with cartilage and bone, but orderly maturation is present in fracture callus and stress fractures	Small round blue cells with regular size, primitive-appearing cells t(11;22)(q24;q12) chromosome rearrangement and CD99+ve	Sheets of giant cells and mononuclear stromal cells	Benign-appearing chondrocytes, without osteoid differentiation Nuclear grooves Chicken wire vascular stroma

Table 5.
Differential diagnosis of conventional osteosarcoma (NOS), fracture callus, Ewing's sarcoma, GCT, and chondroblastoma.

two types of tumor osteoid, early-tumor osteoid, lacelike pattern around tumor cells, and late-tumor osteoid, a mineralized one having an appearance of a woven bone, but an important feature is that tumor osteoid is not rimmed by osteoblasts [16].

6.2 Osteomyelitis

Osteomyelitis is an important cause of morbidity and mortality in children and adults due to acute and chronic bacterial infection. More common sites are the metaphysis and epiphysis of the lower limbs and vertebrae [26–28].

Primary (hematogenous) osteomyelitis is associated with fever and local painful mass and may have fistula formation. A history of recent trauma with open fracture is significant for secondary osteomyelitis. The radiology and MRI are more helpful in the diagnosis of these lesions [26]. The C-reactive protein and erythrocyte sedimentation rate (ESR) are markedly elevated. Biopsy shows necrotic bone, fibrotic marrow, and chronic inflammation with or without an acute inflammatory component. Reactive bone is usually produced as part of an associated periosteal reaction, readily differentiated using histological features [24] (**Table 6**).

6.3 Osteoblastoma

It is a benign osteoid-producing tumor with roughly the same age and sex distribution as osteosarcoma. In conventional radiography, there is a well-defined round expansile mass with central radiolucent zone (>1.5 cm) and a peripheral rim of sclerosis (sclerosis may not be as extensive as in osteoid osteoma). On biopsy, there is an irregular interlacing network of osteoid with prominent osteoblastic rimming and features of woven bone; the differential diagnosis from OS is sometimes difficult when the OS is well differentiated and OB is showing bizarre osteoblasts due to degenerative activities [24] (**Table 4**).

6.4 Aneurysmal bone cyst (ABC)

ABC has the same age range and location as osteosarcoma. It presents with pain and occasional pathological fracture. Secondary aneurysmal bone cysts can be seen in older patients, superimposed on other primary neoplasms. Conventional radiographs show radiolucent expansile bone lesion. MRI shows fluid levels on T2-weighted images. Biopsy can differentiate from telangiectatic osteosarcoma (TOS), which displays obvious histological features of malignancy (marked cellular pleomorphism, high and abnormal mitotic activity) (**Figure 5**) [24, 29] (**Table** 7).

6.5 Fibrous dysplasia (FD)

It is a nonneoplastic intramedullary condition, associated with two forms, monostotic (seen in the ribs, femur, and tibia in young adults) and polyostotic (endocrine dysfunctions). The presentation of polyostotic fibrous dysplasia commonly includes bone deformity and pathological fracture. It has wide age range at presentation and no gender preference. The radiographs show a fusiform expanded swelling with thinning of cortex not associated soft with tissue mass. There are generally no aggressive radiographical features. Pathological fracture may be seen [24].

Microscopically, there are curved and irregularly shaped trabeculae-like fish-hook configuration. These are interspersed in fibrous stroma of variable cellularity. These poorly moralized bony trabeculae have no rimming of osteoblasts, and cartilaginous islands are present in 10% of cases [30].

Features	Osteosarcoma	Osteomyelitis	Langerhans granuloma	Fibrous dysplasia
Site and location	Long bone	Epiphysis (neonates) Metaphysis (children)	Metaphysis or diaphysis	Medulla of diaphysis
Age in years	10–25	Any age, more in children	More common in children 5–15 years	1–30 years > males
Clinical symptoms	Pain	Pain, fever, discharges	Local pain	No pain
Radiology	Radiographically, osteosarcoma is poorly circumscribed with cortical destruction and evidence of periosteal reactive bone Permeative pattern of growth at the periphery	The earliest radiological changes are seen in adjacent soft tissues +/− muscle outlines with swelling and loss or blurring of normal fat planes. An effusion may be seen in an adjacent joint. MRI is more helpful	Multiple lytic lesions with significant periosteal reaction	The conventional radiographs show ground glass appearance with no associated soft tissue mass. There are generally no aggressive radiographical features
Histology	Tumor osteoid is arranged in parallel arrays and separated by a hypocellular fibroblastic stroma. Atypia is common The spindle cells between bony trabeculae instead of fat and hematopoietic tissue as seen in OS Lacks the fibrovascular stroma and osteoblastic rimming of osteoid osteoma May show cartilage component	In acute cases, neutrophils and necrotic bony trabeculae, in TB, granulomas, and in chronic nonspecific cases, lymphocytes and macrophages are more common	There is monoclonal proliferation of Langerhans cells (distinctive cells of monocyte–macrophage lineage) and should be considered a malignancy although its biological behavior is very variable. EM shows Birbeck granules. Express CD1a, S100, HLA-DR	There is large fibrous matrix with scattered curvilinear irregularly shaped trabeculae of immature, inadequately mineralized bone. There is no rimming by osteoblasts GNAS +ve, osteoclastin +ve Run-X-2 +ve, see also (**Table 9**)

Table 6.
Differential diagnosis of osteosarcoma, with osteomyelitis, Langerhans granuloma, and fibrous dysplasia.

It should be differentiated from other bony lesions, cemento-ossifying fibroma (rimming of osteoblast), chondrosarcoma (binucleation), Paget's disease (mosaic pattern bone histologically), non-ossifying fibroma (metaphyseal fibrous defect in tibia with the absence of osteoid), simple bony cyst, and osteofibrous dysplasia/ossifying fibroma (exclusively seen in the tibia almost, with anterior bowing of the bone, in the cortex; rimming is seen around lamellar bony trabeculae) [30].

Some immunomarkers are helpful in the diagnosis of FD. Fibroblastic cells in FD and ossifying fibroma show strong Runx2 expression in the nucleus, while osteocalcin is seen in calcified regions in FD, and G protein genes (GNAS) are positive in extragnathic FD. FD shows GNAS (G protein gene) mutation not seen 15 in other lesions. FD is negative for osteocalcin [31, 32] (**Table 6**).

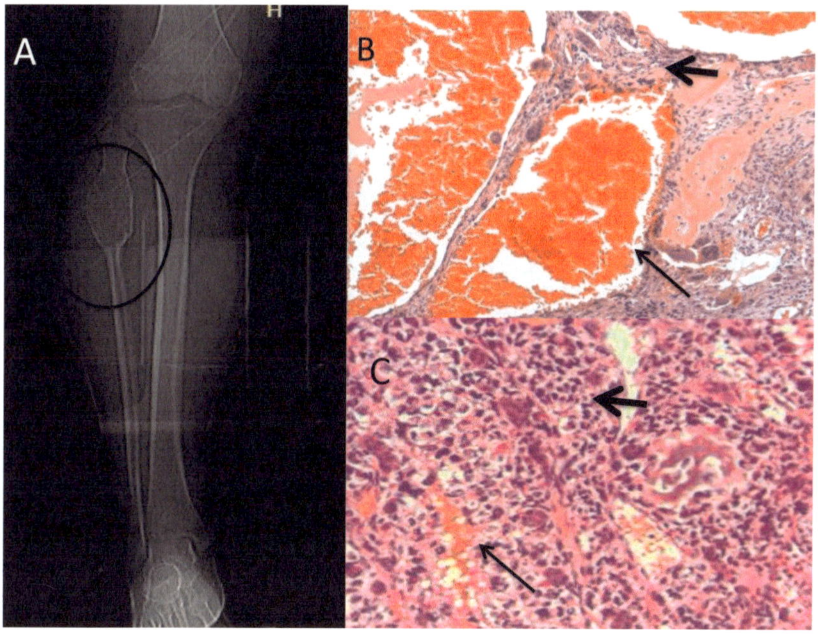

Figure 5.
(A) Radiological examination of telangiectatic osteosarcoma revealing a lytic/expansile, (ring) permeative lesion in the proximal fibula metaphysis with a wide zone of transition and cortical destruction, (B&C) histological examination of the photomicrographs (B; 5X and C; 400X, H&E) blood-filled spaces (thin arrows), separated by septa containing highly malignant cells (small arrows).

6.6 Ewing's sarcoma

It is the second commonest primary malignant bone tumor of the childhood after osteosarcoma. It typically arises from the medullary cavity and invades the Haversian system. Radiologically, It presents as moth-eaten and destructive permeated lucent lesions in the shaft of the long bones. It appears typical onionskin appendence due to periostitis. It may also involve flat bones and appears sclerotic in up to 30% of cases [33].

Same age range and predilection for males. Type II symptoms (e.g., fever, night sweats) are usually seen. Conventional radiographs show a metaphyseal or diaphyseal tumor with a predominantly lytic appearance. No bone matrix is radiographically identified. Onionskin appearance in ES on radiology. MRI shows a large soft tissue mass.

Biopsy shows small round blue cell tumor with no osteoid production. Cytogenetic and/or molecular studies show the typical translocations/molecular aberrations of Ewing sarcoma family of tumors and help rule out small cell osteosarcoma (a rare subtype of osteosarcoma with very little osteoid production). CD 99 is positive in EWS [6, 33] (**Table 5**).

6.7 Chondrosarcoma

It is a cartilage-producing sarcoma with these differences with osteosarcoma. It is most common in patients between 50 and 60 years of age and not seen in less than 20 years. The tumor has a predilection for the pelvic bones and a slower growth rate. Conventional radiographs show a lytic lesion centered in the long bone metaphysis, with a permeative growth pattern scalloping the cortex and showing intra-tumoral calcifications, with a flocculent or ring-shaped appearance. The

Features	Telangiectatic osteosarcoma (TOS)	Conventional OS	Angiosarcoma	ABC	Giant cell tumors
Site and location	Metaphysis	Metaphysis	Not specific	Metaphysis Flat bones, vertebrae, long bones	Metaphysis of epiphysis
Age in years	Mean age 20 years	10–25	Old age	Younger 10–20, slightly more in females	>20 up to 40
Clinical symptoms	Dull pain	Dull pain	No pain	No pain	No pain
Radiology	Lytic bony lesions, geographic bony destruction with wide zone of transition tends to be more common than permeative bony destruction	Sclerotic lesions and cortical destruction	Soft tissue mass	Lytic but demarcated Both processes may have similar presentations and radiographic findings and tend to involve the vertebra CT and MRI show fluid level	Soap bubble appearance
Histology	It is consist of vascular sinusoids surrounded by thin septae, osteoid matrix and cells with significant pleomorphism and high mitotic rate	Malignant osteoblasts and malignant osteoids IHC:SATB2 and AKP are positive, TP53 alteration and MDM2 amplification	Blood vessels are lined by malignant endothelial cells	Small foci of reactive osteoid may be present in aneurysmal bone cysts, which should not be confused with osteoblastoma IHC shows rearrangement of USP6, gene present of Ch 17, t(16;17)(q22;p13). Fusion of USP6 with CDH11	Sheets of giant cells and mononuclear stromal cells. Sometimes, may appear with blood-filled spaces

Note: ABC; Aneurysmal bone cyst, GCT; Giant cell tumors, OS; Osteosarcoma, IHC; Immunohistochemistry, Ch; chromosome.

Table 7.
Differential diagnosis of telangiectatic osteosarcoma (TOS) and, conventional osteosarcoma, angiosarcoma, ABC, and GCT.

cortex is usually thickened with a slightly expanded fusiform appearance, mainly due to the slow permeative growth of the tumor (chronic periosteal reaction). Scalloping of the inner cortex is a radiographic sign worrisome for malignancy. Biopsy is the confirmatory test. Low-grade CS with ossification may mimic OS, but the cartilaginous component in OS, if seen, is always high-grade and malignant osteoids are essential for its diagnosis. Dedifferentiated CS has a well-differentiated benign chondral lesion or chondrosarcoma and sharply juxtaposed with a high-grade non-cartilaginous component; typically, there is an abrupt transition between the two tissue types. The non-cartilaginous component of dedifferentiated chondrosarcoma is generally osteosarcoma, a fibrosarcoma, or a malignant fibrous histiocytoma. Dedifferentiation to leiomyosarcoma, giant cell tumor, and, rarely, clear-cell chondrosarcoma or rhabdomyosarcoma has been reported. Always look the age, site and radiology for help. The S-100 is negative in OS [34].

6.8 Giant cell tumor (GCT) of the bone

The GCT is usually benign and arises from long bone epiphysis and metaphysis. It is rare in vertebrae, but when they occur in a vertebra, the body and not the arch is usually involved [35]. The pathogenesis of GCT is accredited due to overexpression of a tumor necrosis factor receptor (RANK/RANKL) which results in a hyper-proliferation of osteoclasts [16]. Histologically, the GCTs are characterized by the presence of osteoclast-like, giant cells and round-to-oval polygonal mononuclear cells. Frequent mitotic figures in the mononuclear cells may be seen, especially in pregnant women or those on the oral contraceptive pill (due to increased hormone levels) [16, 35]. Important features are given below (**Table 5**).

This lesion is most common in skeletally mature women with closed epiphysis which usually presents with bone pain and sometimes pathological fractures. It involves epiphysis and extends to joint articular cartilage. Conventional radiographs show tumor with an osteolytic appearance located in the epiphysis of long bones, with the distal femur and proximal tibia being the most commonly affected. No doubt it is benign but is locally aggressive. This translates radiographically into the absence of an osteosclerotic rim at its periphery as well as the presence of a soft tissue mass. No bone/osteoid formation is identified. Radiology is soap bubble appearance. Biopsy shows typical appearance of evenly distributed giant cells in a mononuclear stroma. The nuclei of the giant cells resemble the nuclei of the histiocytes. There is atypia or mitosis, potentially malignant with 50% recurrence rate and 10% metastasis [32].

6.9 Primary lymphoma of the bones

These are rare manifestation than secondary lymphoma involving the bone. It is rare, accounting for <5% of bone tumors and <1% of non-Hodgkin lymphoma. It is more common in old age males as compared to OS. The patient presents with type II general symptoms like night sweatings, fever, and weight loss. The conventional radiographs may be normal (tumor cells tend to grow between patient's bony trabeculae with little bone destruction). There may be multiple or single bone involvement. MRI shows focal change in the marrow signal. Bone marrow biopsy is usually the confirmatory test. Flow cytometric studies should be considered in patients suspected of having lymphoma. Leukocyte common antigen (LCA) is positive in lymphomas while negative in OS [24, 36]. Usually it should be differentiated from infections, small cell OS, Ewing's sarcoma, eosinophilic granuloma, and metastatic lesions [36, 37].

6.10 Langerhans cell histiocytosis

It is a multisystem but rare disease. It is associated with a wide and heterogeneous clinical spectrum and extent of multisystem involvement. The age range is 5–15 years, more common in the children and early teens. The males are more affected than females (M/F ratio is 3:2) [38, 39]. It has a predilection for the bones of the skull, the calvarium, but any other bone like the humerus, femur, and ribs can be involved. There is local pain and swelling. Radiographically there are multiple lytic lesions with significant periosteal reaction. Biopsy shows a proliferation of neoplastic Langerhans cells in an inflammatory background [24] (**Table 6**).

6.11 Metastases from other malignancies

Generally it occurs in older age group than osteosarcoma. There is usual history of a primary malignancy known to metastasis to bone, such as breast, lung, thyroid, kidney, and prostate. Conventional radiographs and radionuclide scans usually show osteolytic lesions (rarely osteoblastic) involving multiple bones. CT imaging may reveal other organs affected by metastatic disease. Biopsy usually confirms the diagnosis [35].

7. Special variants of OS with differential diagnosis

7.1 Telangiectatic OS

It is an uncommon variant of OS in the second decade with a mean age of 20 years. It comprises of 2.5–12% of all osteosarcomas. Almost all osteosarcomas have telangiectatic component. In order to diagnose telangiectatic osteosarcoma, there should be more than 90% component with telangiectatic features. It is more common in males like conventional OS (with a ratio of 2:1 for male to female) [24] better than conventional OS [13].

Multiple cyst-like spaces resemble an aneurysmal bone cyst, except that the septa of the cysts contain stromal cells (mononuclear and multinucleated) with cytologically malignant changes. Mitotic figures are present, including atypical forms. Sometimes the malignant stromal cells are floating in the center of the large hemorrhagic cysts; identification of the stromal cells may be difficult, requiring multiple sections. The TOS may arise in other bony diseases like fibrous dysplasia, Paget's disease, or postradiation therapy. Malignant osteoid can be difficult to identify, usually focal and found in a delicate lacelike pattern [24, 40] (**Figure 5** and **Table 7**).

Advice: If the diagnosis of aneurysmal bone cyst is being considered, all tissue should be evaluated histologically for evidence of malignant stroma to rule out telangiectatic osteosarcoma radiological correlation.

7.2 Differential diagnosis of TOS

7.2.1 Aneurysmal bone cyst

The aneurysmal bone cysts are usually seen in young age with slight female preponderance in flat and vertebral areas but may involve long bones. Radiology shows a lucent expansile lesion in the metaphysis of long bones with thin reactive covering of periosteal bone. CT and MRI show some fluid levels in the ABC. Microscopically, thin blood filled spaces. These spaces are not lined by endothelium but only fibroblastic cells are there. The stroma of the ABC may be cellular but typically lacks cytological atypia and atypical mitoses and may contain reactive bone with atypical osteoblasts. Cytologic malignant features and atypical mitoses are absent (**Figure 6**, **Table 7**).

7.2.2 Conventional osteosarcoma

Radiographically, these tumors are not purely lytic. Intramedullary osteosarcoma may contain focal telangiectatic areas, which should not be overinterpreted (**Table 8**).

7.3 Well-differentiated intraosseous low-grade osteosarcoma

The low-grade OS is a rare subtype of osteosarcoma, usually occurring in young adults in their tibia and femur. Microscopically, there may be components of heavy osteoid and fibrocollagenous stroma, and the cells appear benign but with invasion of cortex and surrounding soft tissue. The spindle cells are with mild atypia, marked collagen production, scant atypia, and abundant osteoid production (**Figure 9**). The patients present with pain and swelling in older people. It arises from metaphysis of long bone of lower extremity, while other sites are uncommon. Radiologically, there are irregularly sclerotic lesions with poorly defined sclerotic margins, and mineralized matrix is common (**Figure 7A–C**).

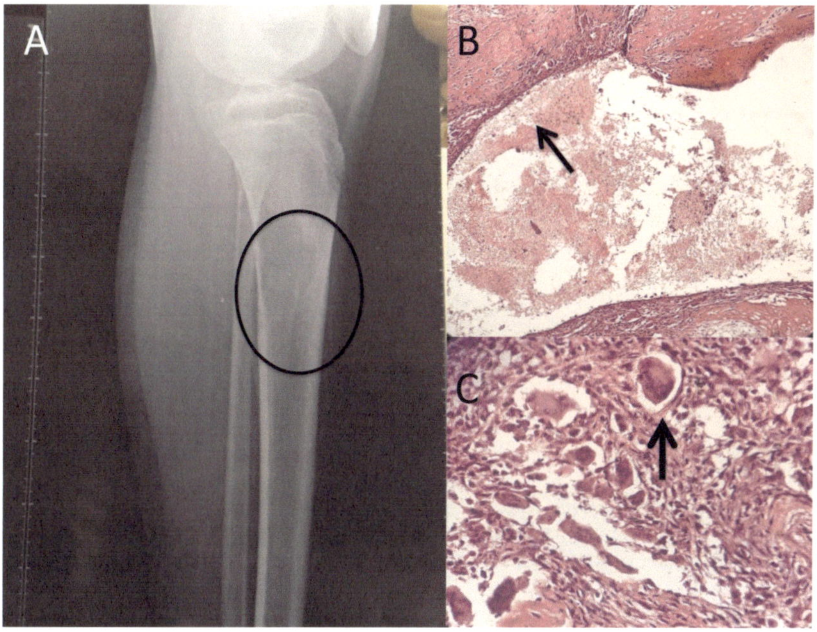

Figure 6.
(A) Radiological examination reveals (ring) homogenous cystic areas (aneurysmal bone cyst) without cortical destructions. (B) Photomicrograph (H&E 10X) revealing cystic lesions (arrow), with giant cells (red arrow) separated by fibrous septa (black arrows), alternating with solid areas and septa lined by fibroblasts, myofibroblasts, and histiocytes but not endothelium (C).

7.4 Differential diagnosis of well-differentiated OS

7.4.1 Chondroblastoma

Chondroblastoma is a rare primary bone tumor of young people that typically arises at the ends of the long bones. Radiologic investigations show a small, circumscribed, lytic lesion. The tumor is characterized histologically by the proliferation of chondroblasts along with areas of mature cartilage, giant cells, and, occasionally, secondary aneurysmal bone cyst formation. Chondroblastoma, however, may also present with atypical features, such as prominent hemosiderin deposition, numerous giant cells, or the presence of a large aneurysmal bone cyst component.

A rare variant of osteosarcoma with CB features may be seen and can be difficult to distinguish from CB, as both tumors can present in young patients as a lytic lesion in an epiphyseal location. Histologically, this OS may reveal small round-oval cells with eosinophilic cytoplasm and scattered giant cells and therefore may cause confusion with CB, especially on a small biopsy specimen. Clues to the appropriate malignant diagnosis include a more aggressive, infiltrative lesion on radiological studies, and the presence of nuclear atypia, atypical mitoses, and/or malignant osteoid production on histologic examination (**Table 5**).

7.4.2 Fibrous dysplasia

It is usually seen in young ages (10–30 years) and more common in males. It is commonly found in metaphysis, diaphysis of ribs, jaw, skull, tibia, and femur. It is locally aggressive tumor and may be monostotic or polyostotic and associated with

Features	Osteosarcoma	MFH	Lymphoma	Osteoblastoma
Site and location	Metaphysis of long bone	Metaphysis of the long bones	Metaphysis	Metaphysis
Age in years	10–25	10 to 60, commonly seen in the second decade	50–60	Younger age and more in females 10–30
Clinical symptoms	Pain	Dull pain but may be associated when arising from other primary bone lesions, like Paget's disease, radiation, giant cell tumor, and bone infarction	Localized pain and swelling	Pain
Radiology	Radiographically, osteosarcoma is poorly circumscribed with cortical destruction and evidence of periosteal reactive bone Permeative pattern of growth at the periphery	Purely osteolytic permeative lesions without a periosteal reaction and without mineralization	The most common is a lytic pattern with permeative bone destruction and a wide zone of transition	Well-defined lytic lesions
Histology	Tumor osteoid is arranged in parallel arrays and separated by a hypocellular fibroblastic stroma. Atypia is common The spindle cells between bony trabeculae instead of fat and hematopoietic tissue as seen in OS Lacks the fibrovascular stroma and osteoblastic rimming of osteoid osteoma May show cartilage component	No extensive osteoid formation. Some osteoid osteogenic sarcomas may have a predominant histologic pattern of malignant fibrous histiocytoma; the presence of osteoid formation requires the diagnosis of osteosarcoma They are heterogeneous fibroblastic tumors formed by poorly differentiated fibroblasts, myofibroblasts, histiocyte-like cells with high degree of pleomorphism and characteristic storiform pattern and also demonstrating bizarre multinucleated giant cells Run-X-2 negative	DLBCL is the most common subtype. The bony pelvis and femur are the most common locations	They manufacture abundant osteoid, but they are not composed of atypical and pleomorphic osteoblasts

DLBCL; Diffuse large B cell lymphoma, MFH; Malignant Fibrous Histiocytoma.

Table 8.
Differential diagnosis of osteosarcoma with malignant fibrous histiocytoma, lymphoma, and osteoblastoma.

endocrine disorders. Radiologically, it is circumscribed radiolucent lesions, within the medullary cavity.

There are irregularly shaped bony trabeculae without rimming of osteoblasts.

The osteoids are of mature woven bones, and irregular in FD, while mature osteoids are present in WDIOS. There is no cortical destruction on X-rays seen in

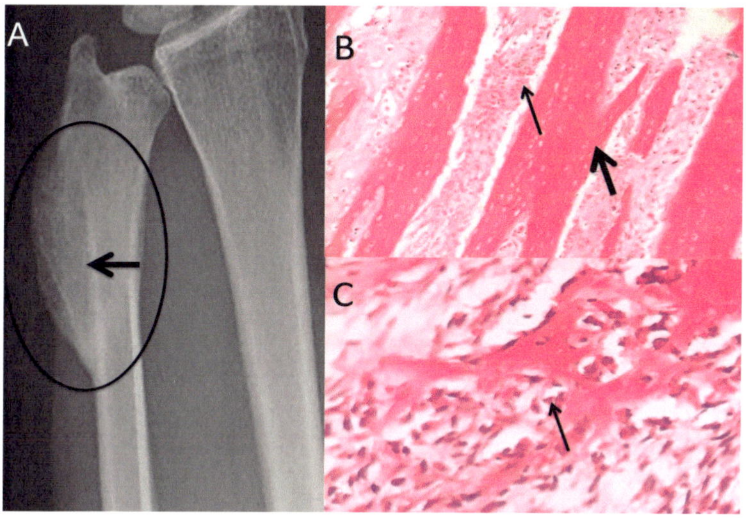

Figure 7.
(A) Radiological examination showing medullary and cortical bone destruction wide zone of transition (ring and arrow), permeative or moth-eaten appearance. (B) Photomicrograph of (10X H&E) of conventional ***intramedullary osteosarcoma*** *and bony osteoid (thick arrow) surrounded by pleomorphic stroma and mitoses (thin arrows) (20X H&E) (C).*

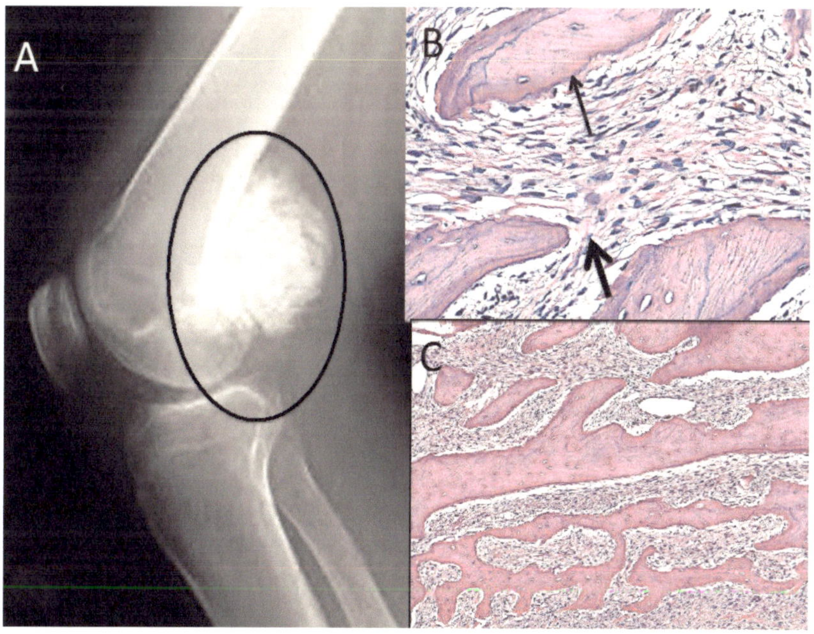

Figure 8.
X-ray of parosteal osteosarcoma (ring) showing surface-attached mass (A). Photomicrograph (H&E 20X) revealing continuously branching bony trabeculae (thick arrow) with spindle cell proliferation of malignant cells (thin arrow) (B and C).

FD, while there are irregularly sclerotic lesions with poorly defined sclerotic margins. The mineralized matrix is common in WDIOS while lacking in FD (**Tables 6** and **9**).

7.4.3 Non-ossifying fibroma (cortical fibrous defect)

Usually seen in young persons, it is a benign lesion. Microscopically, no osteoid and bony trabeculae but only storiform spindle stroma, giant cells, and hemosiderin-laden microphages are seen. Radiologically, these are eccentric sharply defined lytic lesions in metaphyseal cortex in young people.

7.4.4 Parosteal osteosarcoma (PAOS)

This infrequent variant occurs in a juxtacortical position in the metaphyses of long bones and grows very slowly. It grows, as a lobulated mass around the bone shafts as a low-grade malignant bone tumor with well-formed bony trabeculae,

Features	**WD intramedullary OS**	**PAOS**	**COS**	**PEOS**	**Fibrous dysplasia**
Site and location	Metaphysis	Metaphysis	Metaphysis	Metaphysis	Medulla of diaphysis.
Age in years	10–20	10–25	10–25	10–25	1–30 years > males
Clinical symptoms	Pain and swelling, patients older	Dull pain	Dull pain	Dull pain	No pain
Radiology	Irregularly sclerotic lesions with poorly defined sclerotic margins, mineralized matrix common	Radiodense, bosselated, or mushroom-shaped mass arising on the surface of a bone; in long-term lesions, tumor may encircle the bone	Diffuse cortical destruction like Codman's triangle, osteoblastic features	Broad-based surface soft-tissue mass causing extrinsic erosion of thickened underlying diaphyseal cortex and perpendicular periosteal reaction extending into the soft-tissue	The conventional radiographs show ground glass appearance with no associated soft tissue mass. There are generally no aggressive radiographical features
Histology	Heavy osteoid component, fibrocollagenous stroma with minimal atypia	Tumor osteoid is arranged in parallel arrays and separated by a hypocellular fibroblastic stroma that exhibits minimal cytologic atypia and minimal mitotic activity without atypical forms	This is a higher-grade osteosarcoma involving the medullary cavity. Periosteal osteosarcoma does not involve the medullary cavity	Osteosarcoma with prominent cartilaginous component. The cartilage in lobules with peripheral spindling and central bone formation. Malignant osteoid/ bone is present but may be focal	There is large fibrous matrix with scattered curvilinear irregularly shaped trabeculae of immature, inadequately mineralized bone. There is no rimming by osteoblasts differentiating feature from cement-ossifying fibroma. Cartilaginous islands are present in 10%, differentiating feature from chondroblastoma

Note: Well-differentiated intramedullary osteosarcoma (WDIOS), parosteal osteosarcoma (PAOS), fibrous dysplasia (FD), conventional osteosarcoma (COS).

Table 9.
Differential diagnosis of WD intramedullary osteosarcoma, parosteal osteosarcoma, conventional OS, periosteal osteosarcoma, and fibrous dysplasia.

osteoid, variable cartilage, and highly fibrous spindle cell stroma in disorganized manner. In some cases there may be hypocellularity, but there is always mild atypia in the stroma. These tumors have a slight female predominance, with a male-to-female ratio of 1:1.5, and occur predominantly in the third decade. About three fourths of cases involve the distal posterior femur, with the proximal tibia as the second most common site. Clinically it presents as a painless mass of long duration; pain may occur late in the course of this tumor but is not evident initially. Microscopically, there is disorderly arrangement of well-formed bony trabeculae and osteoid and exceptionally osteoclast-like giant cells. There are spindle-shaped stroma with mild atypia and variable amount of cartilage (**Table 9**) compared to conventional OS (**Figure 8** and **Table 9**). Radiodense, bosselated, or mushroom-shaped mass arises on the surface of a bone; in long-term lesions, tumor may encircle the bone [41].

7.5 Differential diagnosis PAOS

7.5.1 Osteochondroma

It is a benign disorder where the medullary spaces contain adipose tissue or marrow hematopoietic tissue with cartilaginous cap. The bony trabeculae are normally arranged as compared to the PAOS.

7.5.2 Myositis ossificans

The myositis ossificans (MO) is distinguished from PAOS by its orderly pattern of maturation. Radiologically, things appear inverse in the MO as compared to PAOS. There is the dense ossification in the center in MO and opaque bone at the periphery, making it eggshell in appearance. Histologically there is zonal arrangement. Maturation toward lamellar bone and marrow adipose tissue begins

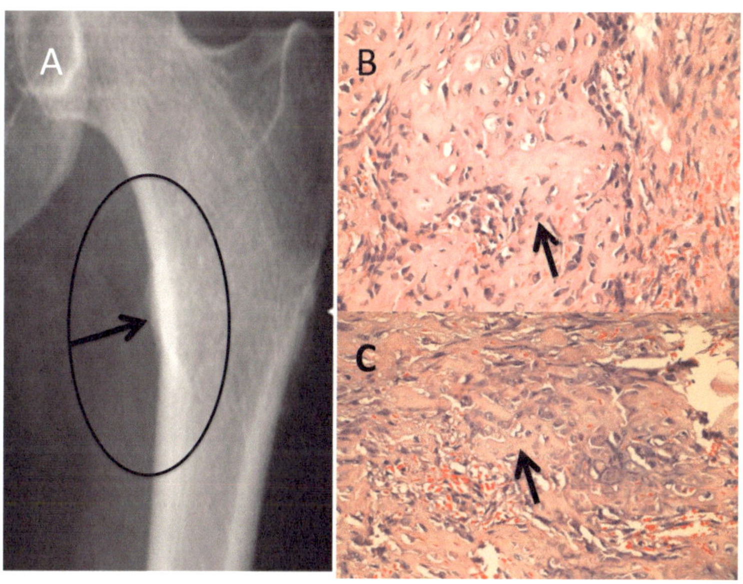

Figure 9.
X-ray of periosteal osteosarcoma (ring) showing broad-based lesion thickening of cortical areas of the femur (A). Photomicrograph (H&E 40X) revealing bony trabeculae with spindle cell proliferation (arrow) of malignant cells and cartilage (red arrow) differentiation (B and C).

peripherally and extends centrally in this proliferative process, which is the reverse in parosteal osteosarcoma [41].

7.5.3 Osteochondroma

The osteochondroma shows continuity of corticomedullary areas of the tumor and the underlying medullary canal, but these features are lacking in PAOS. Medullary spaces contain adipose tissue or marrow hematopoietic tissue, cartilaginous cap.

7.5.4 Periosteal osteosarcoma

Abundant cartilage is present. Higher-grade osseous component and evidence of periosteal reaction.

7.5.5 Periosteal osteosarcoma (PEOS)

This malignant bone tumor is commonly seen in routine biopsies, entirely different from PAOS (juxtacortical OS) despite its similarity with terminology. It arises on surface of long bones (upper tibia and femur). The PEOS affects a slightly older age group (10–20 years) as compared to conventional osteosarcoma. Malignant osteoid must be present, but the predominant pattern of tumor is represented by lobulated chondromatous tissue with cytologic features of grade 2 or 3 chondrosarcoma. Tumor is located on the surface of the bone and may extend into soft tissue. The lesions are limited to the cortex and rarely invade the medullary cavity. The tumor appears perpendicular to the shaft. Sometimes high-grade anaplastic sarcomatous spindle cell component may separate lobules of the malignant chondroid component [24] (**Figure 9** and **Table 10**) [20, 42].

7.6 Differential diagnosis of PEOS

7.6.1 Periosteal chondroma

It is usually smaller and better defined and composed of benign chondroid tissue and does not contain malignant tumor osteoid [24].

7.6.2 Periosteal chondrosarcoma

Radiographically, it contains "popcorn" calcifications, and histologically, it is a low-grade chondrosarcoma containing no tumor osteoid [20, 24].

7.6.3 Parosteal osteosarcoma

Radiographically, this tumor is more radiodense, and histologically this is a low-grade malignant fibro-osseous tumor without chondroid differentiation [20, 24].

7.6.4 Conventional intramedullary osteosarcoma

This is a higher-grade osteosarcoma involving the medullary cavity. Periosteal osteosarcoma does not involve the medullary cavity [24].

DOI: http://dx.doi.org/10.5772/intechopen.85190

Features	PAOS	COS	PEOS	Osteochondroma	Myositis ossificans	Parosteal lipoma
Site and location	Metaphysis	Metaphysis	Metaphysis	Metaphyseal	NOS	NOS
Age in years	10–25	10–25	10–25	10–30	Any age	Any age
Clinical symptoms	Dull pain	Dull pain	Dull pain	No pain	Pain	No pain
Radiology	Radiodense, bosselated, or mushroom-shaped mass arising on the surface of a bone; in long-term lesions, tumor may encircle the bone	Diffuse cortical destruction like Codman's triangle, osteoblastic features	Broad-based surface soft-tissue mass causing extrinsic erosion of thickened underlying diaphyseal cortex and perpendicular periosteal reaction extending into the soft-tissue	Metaphyseal lesions grow in direction opposite to adjacent joint. Cortex and medulla are continuous with underlying bone		Lytic lesions without bony destructions
Histology	Tumor osteoid is arranged in parallel arrays and separated by a hypocellular fibroblastic stroma that exhibits minimal cytologic atypia and minimal mitotic activity without atypical forms	This is a higher-grade osteosarcoma involving the medullary cavity. Periosteal osteosarcoma does not involve the medullary cavity	Osteosarcoma with prominent cartilaginous component. The cartilage in lobules with peripheral spindling and central bone formation. Little no. of mitosis Malignant osteoid/bone is present but may be focal	Bony trabeculae appear normal	Orderly maturation, not attached to underlying bone; more active histologically	Lipocytes, no osteoid

Note: Parosteal Osteosarcoma, PAOS; Conventional Osteosarcoma, COS; Periosteal osteosarcoma, PEOS.

Table 10.
Differential diagnosis of parosteal osteosarcoma, conventional osteosarcoma, periosteal osteosarcoma, osteochondroma, myositis ossificans, and parosteal lipoma.

7.6.5 High-grade surface osteosarcoma

It lacks cartilaginous differentiation. Osteoid component is pleomorphic and high grade [12, 13].

8. High-grade surface osteosarcoma

This is a high-grade osteosarcoma with similar histological features to those of conventional intramedullary osteosarcoma. The tumor grows on the surface and lacks significant medullary involvement. Radiographically it mimics periosteal osteosarcoma, except it has cumulus cloud-like patterns of mineralization. It is a large, lobulated surface mass with variable consistency ranging from soft to firm and may contain hemorrhagic areas. It should not significantly involve the medullary region [13, 24].

8.1 Differential diagnosis of high-grade OS

8.1.1 Dedifferentiated parosteal osteosarcoma

It usually has residual low-grade malignant fibroblastic stromal component. Parosteal osteosarcoma lacks high-grade anaplastic appearance [12, 24].

8.1.2 Conventional intramedullary osteosarcoma

Significant medullary component (minimal medullary component in a high-grade surface osteosarcoma) [24].

8.1.3 Low-grade central osteosarcoma

It is a large, poorly marginated intramedullary mass that either is sclerotic or exhibits trabeculations and histologically similar to parosteal osteosarcoma [12, 24].

9. Summary

Osteosarcoma (OS) is a high-grade malignancy of the bone with high-mortality rate. The exact cause of the condition is unknown, and presently, it is not possible to prevent an osteosarcoma occurrence. It is mainly divided into two types, primary and secondary, based on etiology, while based on where they occur, osteosarcoma is classified as medullary osteosarcoma (occurring in the bone cavity) and surface osteosarcoma (occurring on the bone surface). OS has a bimodal age distribution, having the first peak during adolescence and the second peak in older adulthood, while a little bit more common in males. Some genetic mutations, like mutation of RB and P53 genes, are associated with osteosarcoma. Radiation affected persons, patients of Paget's disease of the bone, fibrous dysplasia, osteoblastoma, Ollier disease, and chemotherapy, are other conditions and disorders that are thought to be associated with Osteosarcomas. The tumor grows slowly in the initial phase of the tumors and may be asymptomatic. Then tumors grow at a moderate rate, and then they suddenly start to rapidly progress. Pathological fractures are commonly seen in long bones.

Three parameters are used for its diagnosis, physical examination with medical history, radiological support (X-rays, CT, MRI), and biopsy for microscopic examination. To approach the remedy of patient, grading and staging with good differential diagnosis are very important to save the life of the patient.

Conflict of interest

None.

Source of support

Nil.

Author details

Mulazim Hussain Bukhari[1]*, Samina Qamar[2] and Farwa Batool[3]

1 Head of Pathology Department, UCMD, University of Lahore, Pakistan

2 King Edward Medical University, Lahore, Pakistan

3 Faisal Abad Medical University, Faisal Abad, Pakistan

*Address all correspondence to: mulazim.husain@gmail.com

References

[1] Dorfman H, Vanel D, Czerniak B, Park Y, Kotz R, Unni K. WHO Classification of Tumours of Bone: Introduction. 2013 [226]. Available from: https://www.iarc.fr/en/publications/pdfs-online/pat-gen/bb5/bb5-classifbone.pdf

[2] Ghadah Al Saanna G, Bovée J, Hornick J, Alexander Lazar A. A review of the WHO classification of tumours of soft tissue and bone. In: Bruce S, Beverly S, editors. The Electronic Sarcoma Update Newsletter (ESUN). NY;USA: Liddy Shriver; 2013

[3] Murphey MD. World Health Organization classification of bone and soft tissue tumors: Modifications and implications for radiologists. Seminars in Musculoskeletal Radiology. 2007; **11**(3):201-214

[4] Chaudhry J, Rawal SY, Anderson KM, Rawal YB. Cancellous osteoma of the maxillary tuberosity: Case report. General Dentistry. 2009;**57**(4): 427-429

[5] Mannava S, Sundaram M. Fibrous dysplasia, osteofibrous dysplasia, and adamantinoma. In: Davico A, Sundaram M, James S, editors. Imaging of Bone Tumors and Tumor-Like Lesions. Medical Radiology. Berlin, Heidelberg: Springer; 2007. pp. 411-424

[6] Greenspan A, Jundt G, Remagen W. Differential Diagnosis in Orthopaedic Oncology. 2nd ed. Philadelphia: Lippincott Williams & Wilkins; 2007

[7] Kaiser MS, Rahman W, Hossain M, Siddiquee TH, Hossain MT, Das KP, et al. Evaluation of outcome of surgical excision of the nidus of osteoid osteoma of long bone. Mymensingh Medical Journal: MMJ. 2014;**23**(4): 686-694

[8] Burgener FA, Kormano M, Pudas T. Bone and Joint Disorders: Differential Diagnosis in Conventional Radiology. New York: Thieme Publishers; 2006. pp. 872

[9] Elstrom JA, Virkus WW, Pankovich A. Handbook of Fractures. 3rd ed. McGraw-Hill Education; 2006

[10] Atesok KI, Alman BA, Schemitsch EH, Peyser A, Mankin H. Osteoid osteoma and osteoblastoma. The Journal of the American Academy of Orthopaedic Surgeons. 2011;**19**(11): 678-689

[11] Jambhekar NA, Desai S, Khapake D. Osteoblastoma: A study of 12 cases. Indian Journal of Pathology & Microbiology. 2006;**49**(4):487-490

[12] Mills S, Greenson J, Hornick J, Longacre T, Reuter V. Sternberg's Diagnostic Surgical Pathology. 6th ed. NY; USA: Wolters Kluwer; 2012

[13] Roasi J. Ackerman's Surgical Pathology. 10th ed. NY; USA: Mosby; 2011. p. 1703

[14] Baker AC, Rezeanu L, Klein MJ, Pitt MJ, Buecker P, Hersh JH, et al. Aggressive osteoblastoma: A case report involving a unique chromosomal aberration. International Journal of Surgical Pathology. 2010;**18**(3):219-224

[15] Harrington C, Accurso BT, Kalmar JR, Iwenofu OH, Agrawal A, Allen CM, et al. Aggressive osteoblastoma of the maxilla: A case report and review of the literature. Head and Neck Pathology. 2011;**5**(2):165-170

[16] Kumar V, Abbas AK, Fausto N. Robbins and Cotran Pathologic Basis of Disease. 9th ed. NY: Elsevier Saunders; 2016. p. 776

[17] Shaikh AB, Li F, Li M, He B, He X, Chen G, et al. Present advances and

future perspectives of molecular targeted therapy for osteosarcoma. International Journal of Molecular Sciences. 2016;**17**(4):506-511

[18] Greenspan A. Orthopedic Imaging: A Practical Approach. NY: Lippincott Williams & Wilkins; 2004. pp. 982

[19] Knipe H, Gaillard F. Osteosarcoma: Radiopaedia.org. Available from: http://radiopaedia.org/articles/osteosarcoma

[20] Yarmish G, Klein MJ, Landa J, Lefkowitz RA, Hwang S. Imaging characteristics of primary osteosarcoma: Nonconventional subtypes. Radiographics. 2010;**30**(6):1653-1672

[21] Xie GP, Song HJ, Jiang N, Qin CH, Wang L, Xu SY, et al. Periosteal osteosarcoma and Marfan's syndrome: A case report and literature review. Oncology Letters. 2016;**11**(1):311-315

[22] Siddiqui YS, Sherwani M, Khan AQ, Zahid M, Abbas M, Asif N. Neglected orthopedic oncology—causes, epidemiology and challenges for management in developing countries. Indian Journal of Cancer. 2015;**52**(3): 325-329

[23] Limmahakhun S, Pothacharoen P, Theera-Umpon N, Arpornchayanon O, Leerapun T, Luevitoonvechkij S, et al. Relationships between serum biomarker levels and clinical presentation of human osteosarcomas. Asian Pacific Journal of Cancer Prevention: APJCP. 2011;**12**(7):1717-1722

[24] Gattuso G, Reddy V, David O, Spitz D, Meryl H, Haber. Bone tumors. In: Differential Diagnosis in Surgical Pathology. 2nd ed. Pheladelphia; PA, USA: Saunders; Elsevier; 2009. p. 336

[25] Jovanovic N, Ristovska N, Bogdanovic Z, Petronijevic M, Opalic J, Plecas D. Diagnosis and treatment of rib fracture during spontaneous vaginal delivery. Srpski Arhiv za Celokupno Lekarstvo. 2013;**141**(7–8):528-531

[26] Lee YJ, Sadigh S, Mankad K, Kapse N, Rajeswaran G. The imaging of osteomyelitis. Quantitative Imaging in Medicine and Surgery. 2016;**6**(2): 184-198

[27] Lew DP, Waldvogel FA. Osteomyelitis. Lancet (London, England). 2004;**364**(9431):369-379

[28] Jaramillo D. Infection: Musculoskeletal. Pediatric Radiology. 2011;**41**(Suppl 1):S127-S134

[29] Kapila R, Sharma R, Sohal YS, Singh D, Singh S. Primary epiphyseal aneurysmal bone cyst of distal ulna. Journal of Orthopaedic Case Reports. 2015;**5**(4):85-87

[30] Fitzpatrick KA, Taljanovic MS, Speer DP, Graham AR, Jacobson JA, Barnes GR, et al. Imaging findings of fibrous dysplasia with histopathologic and intraoperative correlation. AJR American Journal of Roentgenology. 2004;**182**(6):1389-1398

[31] Iida S, Kishino M, Sakai T, Ishida H, Okura M, Toyosawa S, et al. Multiple osseous dysplasia arising from impacted teeth: Report of a case associated with odontogenic lesions. Journal of Oral Pathology & Medicine. 2006;**35**(7): 402-406

[32] Toyosawa S, Yuki M, Kishino M, Ogawa Y, Ueda T, Murakami S, et al. Ossifying fibroma vs fibrous dysplasia of the jaw: Molecular and immunological characterization. Modern Pathology. 2007;**20**(3):389-396

[33] Chen C, Borker R, Ewing J, Tseng WY, Hackshaw MD, Saravanan S, et al. Epidemiology, treatment patterns, and outcomes of metastatic soft tissue sarcoma in a community-based oncology network. Sarcoma. 2014;**2014**: 145764

[34] Schneiderman BA, Kliethermes SA, Nystrom LM. Survival in Mesenchymal Chondrosarcoma varies based on age and tumor location: A survival analysis of the SEER database. Clinical Orthopaedics and Related Research. 2017;**475**(3):799-805

[35] Murphey MD, Nomikos GC, Flemming DJ, Gannon FH, Temple HT, Kransdorf MJ. From the archives of AFIP. Imaging of giant cell tumor and giant cell reparative granuloma of bone: Radiologic-pathologic correlation. Radiographics. 2001;**21**(5):1283-1309

[36] Lim CY, Ong KO. Imaging of musculoskeletal lymphoma. Cancer Imaging. 2013;**13**(4):448-457

[37] Maruyama D, Watanabe T, Beppu Y, Kobayashi Y, Kim SW, Tanimoto K, et al. Primary bone lymphoma: A new and detailed characterization of 28 patients in a single-institution study. Japanese Journal of Clinical Oncology. 2007;**37**(3):216-223

[38] Arceci RJ, Hann IM, Smith OP, Hoffbrand AV. Pediatric Hematology. Wiley; 2006

[39] Gianfreda D, Musetti C, Nicastro M, Maritati F, Cobelli R, Corradi D, et al. Erdheim-Chester disease as a mimic of IgG4-related disease: A case report and a review of a single-center cohort. Medicine. 2016;**95**(21):e3625

[40] Weiss A, Khoury JD, Hoffer FA, Wu J, Billups CA, Heck RK, et al. Telangiectatic osteosarcoma: The St. Jude Children's Research Hospital's experience. Cancer. 2007;**109**(8): 1627-1637

[41] Donmez FY, Tuzun U, Basaran C, Tunaci M, Bilgic B, Acunas G. MRI findings in parosteal osteosarcoma: Correlation with histopathology. Diagnostic and Interventional Radiology (Ankara, Turkey). 2008;**14**(3):142-152

[42] Murphey MD, Jelinek JS, Temple HT, Flemming DJ, Gannon FH. Imaging of periosteal osteosarcoma: Radiologic-pathologic comparison. Radiology. 2004;**233**(1):129-138

Section 3

Basic Science and Translational Treatments

Chapter 3

Long Noncoding RNAs in Osteosarcoma: Mechanisms and Potential Clinical Implications

Christos Valavanis and Gabriela Stanc

Abstract

Long noncoding RNAs (lncRNAs) are noncoding transcripts consisting of a diverse class of long RNAs of more than 200 nucleotides in length. Recent studies have shown that lncRNAs are involved in cell signal transduction pathways, cell cycle and cell death regulation, chromatin remodeling, and gene expression regulation at the transcriptional and posttranscriptional levels. They are also involved in the metastatic process of different types of tumors, such as urothelial carcinoma, colon carcinoma, breast carcinoma, lung carcinoma, and hepatocellular carcinoma. In addition, lncRNAs demonstrate precise expression patterns in specific tissues and cells and therefore play important roles in cell differentiation and tissue development. In this chapter, we review the molecular mechanisms of lncRNA cell functions and their involvement in the pathogenesis, progression, and metastasis of osteosarcoma, a rare bone tumor of childhood and adolescence. We also review emerging clinical implications of lncRNA use as potential prognostic biomarkers and therapeutic targets, as well as their putative involvement in drug resistance, in osteosarcoma progression, and in therapeutic interventions.

Keywords: lncRNAs, osteosarcoma, pathogenesis, prognosis, metastasis, drug resistance

1. Introduction

Osteosarcoma is a rare malignant tumor and the most frequent primary malignant tumor of the bone affecting most often young people in childhood and adolescence [1–3]. It is of mesenchymal histogenetic origin and is characterized by the production of osteoid and fibrous stroma. It has a tendency to be highly anaplastic with cytological pleomorphism consisting of cells of epithelioid, spindle, ovoid, or giant multinucleated appearance and in most cases a mixture of them [4]. It is genetically unstable and exhibits structural chromosomal alterations [5–8]. It represents different pathological entities based on clinical, radiological, and histopathological features. Depending on histopathological features, osteosarcoma displays different subtypes, the most common among them are osteoblastic osteosarcoma, chondroblastic osteosarcoma, and fibroblastic osteosarcoma. Less frequent are telangiectatic osteosarcoma, small cell osteosarcoma, low-grade osteosarcoma, high-grade osteosarcoma, parosteal osteosarcoma, and periosteal osteosarcoma [4, 9–11].

Its incidence is about three to five cases per million population every year worldwide with a propensity of aggressive biological behavior, local infiltrating growth, and distant metastasis [1–3]. About 10–25% of patients are diagnosed with pulmonary metastasis due to hematogenous dissemination, which is the main cause of osteosarcoma mortality [12–14].

Despite its high mortality rates, the combination of ablative resection surgery with chemotherapy or/and radiation therapy has elevated the cure rates of local tumor from less than 20% during 1960s to 65–75% at present days [12–17]. However, patients with disseminated disease demonstrate a 5-year survival rate around 11–30% due to resistance to chemotherapeutic regimens [16–18]. Therefore, developing multimodal more effective treatments along with precise prognostic and preventive biomarkers is imperative, and efforts are on the way to better understand the molecular mechanisms involved in osteosarcoma pathogenesis and define new therapeutic targets.

Recent studies have shown that molecules belonging to the nonprotein-coding transcriptome may play essential roles in a wide range of biological processes [19–21]. These molecules belong to the vast family of nonprotein-coding RNAs which can be classified according to their size or function in two classes: the short noncoding RNAs (sncRNAs) and the long noncoding RNAs (lncRNAs) [22, 23].

Short noncoding RNAs, with a length less than 200 nucleotides, such as microRNAs (miRNAs), transfer RNAs, small interfering RNAs (siRNAs), piwi-interacting RNAs, and some ribosomal RNAs, are estimated to be, till now, about 2500 different types. They are involved in gene expression regulation and have been demonstrated to play important roles in cancer development, progression, and chemoresistance of different tumors including osteosarcoma [22, 23].

On the other hand, lncRNAs are noncoding transcripts consisting of a diverse and heterogeneous class of long RNAs of more than 200 nucleotides –100 kb in length lacking the Kozak consensus sequence and without open reading frame. Their transcription is processed through RNA polymerase II and is regulated by the transcriptional activators of the nucleosome remodeling complex SWI/SNF [23–26]. They are divided in different categories such as intronic lncRNAs, intergenic lncRNAs, UTR-associated lncRNAs, bidirectional lncRNAs, promoter-associated lncRNAs, sense lncRNAs, and antisense lncRNAs [27, 28]. They participate in vital biological processes, such as cell signal transduction, cell cycle and cell death regulation, chromatin remodeling, transcriptional and posttranscriptional processing, as well as in epigenetic gene regulation. They can act as decoys to compete with different proteins, function as sponge to a large number of microRNAs, and interact with RNA-binding proteins. In addition, lncRNAs demonstrate precise expression patterns in specific tissues and cells and therefore play important roles in cell differentiation and tissue development. [29–31]. LncRNA misregulation has been implicated in cancer development, metastatic process, and drug resistance of different types of tumors, such as urothelial carcinoma, colon carcinoma, breast carcinoma, and hepatocellular carcinoma. Aberrant expression of lncRNAs has been seen in different human tumors, an observation that might be exploited for diagnostic, prognostic, preventive, or therapeutic purposes [32–41]. Some of these lncRNAs have also been reported to play a crucial role in osteosarcoma pathogenesis and metastatic process as well as in chemotherapy drug resistance. Thus, they are considered candidate molecules as prognostic or preventive biomarkers and/or novel therapeutic targets [42–47].

In this chapter, we review the molecular mechanisms of lncRNA cell functions and their involvement in the pathogenesis, progression, and metastasis of osteosarcoma. We also review emerging clinical implications of lncRNA use as potential prognostic biomarkers and therapeutic targets, as well as their putative involvement in drug resistance, in osteosarcoma progression, and in therapeutic interventions.

2. LncRNAs and signal transduction pathways in osteosarcoma

Osteosarcomagenesis is initiated in bone epiphyseal growth plates with rapid turnover during childhood and adolescence and has also been observed in high incidence in patients affected by Paget's disease, a pathological entity characterized by excessive osteoid formation and breakdown. These findings suggest that molecular disturbances in osteoblast proliferation and differentiation are involved in osteosarcoma pathogenesis through dysregulation of major signal transduction pathways and osteogenic transcriptional factors [4, 42–47]. Several major signal transduction pathways, mainly Wnt/β-catenin, bone morphogenetic protein (BMP), Hedgehog, HIF1α, Notch, PI3K/Akt, JNK and NF-κB pathways are implicated in osteosarcoma development and metastatic progression [48–50].

The canonical Wnt/β-catenin pathway, which plays a crucial role in osteoblast differentiation, has been found to lead to osteoblast proliferation and suppression of osteogenic differentiation in adult mesenchymal cells through expression of Wnt3a [51–54]. Moreover, aberrations of Wnt signaling pathway have been associated with osteosarcoma tumorigenesis and osteosarcoma drug resistance through upregulation of factors, such as c-Met, leading to stem-cell phenotypes [4, 55–58]. LncRNA H19 has been found to increase Wnt signaling through epigenetical regulation of the Wnt pathway antagonist NKD1 via EZH2 recruitment [59]. Wnt pathway is also activated through TCF7 whose expression is triggered by the recruitment of SWI/SNF nucleosome remodeling complex to the TCF7 promoter by lncTCF7 [60, 61].

Hedgehog (Hh) signaling pathway plays a crucial role during vertebrate embryogenesis acting as a morphogen and mitogen in different tissue development including bone morphogenesis [62–66].

Dysregulation of Hh signaling pathway has been demonstrated to contribute to promigratory effects in osteoblastic osteosarcoma and is related to poor prognosis [67, 68]. Moreover Hedgehog signaling is upregulated in osteosarcoma leading to overexpression of oncogenic yes-associated protein 1(Yap1) which in turn induces the aberrant expression of lncRNA H19 [69].

Bone morphogenetic protein (BMP) signaling pathways synergistically act with Runx2 factor, the most important regulator of bone development, leading to the induction of many terminal differentiation factors and eventually to osteogenic commitment of mesenchymal stem cells. This signaling cascade is initiated by BMP ligand heterodimers (BMPR I and II) binding through Smad and mitogen-activated protein kinase (MAPK) phosphorylation [70–73]. Suppression of osteoblast differentiation has been observed, in one study, after BMP2 treatment of C3H10T1/2 MSCs by downregulation of mouselncRNA0231 and EGFR via Runx2 and osterix regulation [74]. In another study, anti-differentiation lncRNA (ANCR) has been found to suppress osteoblastogenesis through inhibition of Runx2 expression. ANCR interacts with the enhancer of zeste homolog 2 (EZH2); this interaction leads to H3K27me3 catalysis in Runx2 promoter resulting in inhibition of Runx2 expression [75]. Bone morphogenetic protein (BMP) signaling pathways play also an important role in osteosarcoma through RhoA-ROCK-LIMK2 by promoting invasion and metastasis [76, 77].

HIF1α expression levels are elevated in osteosarcoma tissues and are associated with poorer prognosis. Moreover, HIF1α signaling pathway is implicated in osteosarcoma cell invasion through induction of VEGF-A expression [78, 79]. A novel lncRNA, hypoxia-inducible factor-2α (HIF-2α) promoter upstream transcript (HIF2PUT) has been demonstrated to regulate the expression of HIF-2α in osteosarcoma stem cells. Overexpression of HIF2PUT significantly inhibited cell proliferation and migration of MG63 osteosarcoma cells, while HIF2PUT knockdown led to the opposite effect [80].

LncRNA hypoxia-inducible factor 1α-antisense 1 (HIF1α-AS1) is another lncRNA involved in osteoblast differentiation. HIF1α-AS1 expression is repressed by overexpression of histone deacetylase sirtuin 1 (SIRT1), a regulator of osteoblastogenesis, and lower levels of SIRT1 expression lead to upregulation of HIF1α-AS1 in bone marrow stem cells resulting in the activation of osteoblastogenesis [81].

Other studies have also shown the involvement of Notch and JNK signaling pathways in osteosarcoma proliferation, metastasis, angiogenesis, and stemness-associated factors [82, 83].

The phosphatidylinositol 3-kinase PI3K/Akt pathway is considered one of the most critical pathways in osteosarcoma pathogenesis regulating osteosarcoma cell proliferation, invasion, metastasis, and drug sensitivity or resistance [84, 85].

A large number of lncRNAs has been found to be differentially expressed in osteosarcoma either with oncogenic or tumor suppressive activity. Particularly, in a study by Li et al., 25,733 lncRNAs were detected, including 403 constitutively upregulated in 34 pathways and 798 constitutively downregulated in 32 pathways (twofold, $P < 0.05$) [86]. Among them metastasis-associated lung adenocarcinoma transcript 1 (MALAT-1), a lncRNA involved in regulating the recruitment of pre-mRNA-splicing factors to transcription sites, is overexpressed in osteosarcoma, and its expression level is highly related to the metastatic potential of the tumor. In another study, Dong et al. also found that MALAT-1 acts through the PI3K/Akt pathway to promote osteosarcoma cell proliferation, migration, invasion, and pulmonary metastasis [87]. MALAT-1 knockdown or siRNA interference experiments, carried out by Dong et al. and Cai et al., respectively, showed that MALAT1 inhibition suppressed osteosarcoma cell proliferation and metastasis via the PI3K/Akt and RhoA/ROCK signaling pathway by decreasing the expression levels of proliferating cell nuclear antigen (PCNA), Act and phosphorylated PI3Kp85α, as well as MMP-9 metalloproteinase [87, 88].

Another lncRNA, named P50-associated COX-2 extragenic RNA (PACER), has been found to be overexpressed in osteosarcoma clinical specimens and cell lines. PACER has oncogenic effects in osteosarcoma functioning by activating COX-2 gene via the NF-κB signaling cascade [89]. Deregulated NF-κB has been linked to osteosarcoma cell proliferation and metastatic process, and expression of NF-κB has been observed to have clinical value in osteosarcoma patients [90, 91].

3. LncRNAs and regulation of cell growth/proliferation in osteosarcoma

Recent studies have demonstrated the involvement of lncRNAs in cell growth and proliferation of osteosarcoma. Aberrant expression of lncRNAs is implicated in osteosarcoma tumorigenesis through overexpression of oncogenic lncRNAs and inhibition of tumor suppressive lncRNAs [42–44, 92]. These lncRNAs are summarized in **Table 1** along with their function and mechanisms.

3.1 Oncogenic lncRNAs

In recent years, a significant number of oncogenic lncRNAs such as 91H, HULC, FGFR3-AS1, MALAT1, BCAR4, HIF2PUT, TUG1, UCA1, HOTTIP, and HOTAIR have been identified to be implicated in cell growth and proliferation of osteosarcoma.

lncRNA	Chr. locus	Transcript length	Expression	Function	Mechanisms	Refs
91H (H19)	11p15.5	2.3 kb	Upregulated	• Oncogenic • Promotes cell proliferation • Reduced levels • Promote apoptosis	• IGF2 transcriptional regulation • Imprinted gene • miR-141 overexpression leads to OS • Apoptosis through suppression of H19	[94, 95, 197]
BANCR	9q21.11	693 bp	Upregulated	• Promotes tumor growth, invasion, and metastasis	—	[198]
BCAR4	16p13.13	118 bp	Upregulated	• Oncogenic • Promotes cell proliferation	• Activation of GLI2-dependent gene transcription	[104, 105]
DANCR (ANCR)	4q12	855 bp	Upregulated	• Oncogenic • Suppresses osteogenic differentiation • Promotes cell proliferation and metastasis	• Decoy for miR-335-5p and miR-1972 • Inhibits Runx2 expression • Interacts with enhancer of EZH2 • Regulates the expression of p21, CDK2, and CDK4	[100, 101, 207]
FGFR3-AS1	4p16.3	—	Upregulated	• Oncogenic • Promotes cell proliferation	• Increases FGFR3 mRNA stability • Increases FGFR3 expression	[107]
HIF2PUT	2p21		Upregulated	• Oncogenic	• Involvement in HIF-2a and stemness-related genes (Oct4, Sox, CD44) expression	[80, 112]
HOTAIR	12q13.13	2337 bp	Upregulated	• Oncogenic • Promotes cell proliferation, invasion, and metastasis	• Inhibits gene expression through histone H3K27 trimethylation by binding PRC2 and LSD1/CoREST/REST complexes • Upregulation of MMP-2 and MMP-9	[118, 119, 207]
HOTTIP	7p15.2	4.6 kb	Upregulated	• Oncogenic • Promotes cell proliferation, invasion, and metastasis	• Regulates EMT-related molecules (E-cadherin, Snail1, Slug), RNPs, and HOXA genes	[121, 126, 127]
HULC	6p24.3	500 bp	Upregulated	• Oncogenic • Promotes cell proliferation and invasion	• Sponge for miR-200a-3p, miR-9, miR107	[135, 136]
loc285194	3q13.31	2105 bp	Downregulated	• Tumor suppressive • Loss leads to osteoblast proliferation	• Regulation of cell cycle and cell death genes • Regulation of VEGF1 transcription • Regulated by p53 • Represses miR-211	[171, 173, 174]

lncRNA	Chr. locus	Transcript length	Expression	Function	Mechanisms	Refs
lncRNA-ATB	14q11.2	2.4 kb	Upregulated	• Promotes cell proliferation, invasion, and metastasis	• Activated by TGFβ • Enhances EMT • Inhibits miR-200s • Upregulates ZEB1/ZEB2–miR200s target genes	[208, 209, 211, 212]
MALAT-1 (NEAT-2)	11q13.1	8.7 kb	Upregulated	• Oncogenic • Promotes cell proliferation, invasion, and metastasis • Inhibits apoptosis	• Acts through PI3K/Akt and RhoA/ROCK pathways • Competes with miR-376a • Promotes TGFa upregulation • Regulated by Myc-6 • Upregulates MMP-9 and HDAC4 • Decoy for miR-140-5p	[87, 143, 144, 199]
MFI2	3q29	951 bp	Upregulated	• Oncogenic • Promotes cell proliferation and migration	• Enhances FOXP4 expression	[166]
MEG3	14q32.3	1.6 kb	Downregulated	• Tumor suppressor	• Implicated in Wnt/β-catenin pathway • Regulated by lncRNA EWSAT1	[186, 221]
NKILA		2.5 kb	Downregulated	• Promotes invasion and metastasis	• Regulates NF-κB activity through interaction with IκBα	[214]
ODRUL	16q24.1	319 bp	Upregulated	• Promotes invasion and metastasis	• Competes with miR-3182 • Upregulates MMP2	[217]
PACER	1q31.1	793 bp	Upregulated	• Promotes cell proliferation, invasion, and metastasis	• NF-Kb-dependent upregulation of COX-2 • Regulated by CTCF	[89]
SNHG12	1p35.3	1.3 kb	Upregulated	• Oncogenic • Promotes cell proliferation, invasion, and metastasis	• Increases angiomotin expression • Upregulation of Notch2 • Sponge for miR-195-p2 • Upregulation of MMP-2 and MMP-9	[167, 168]
TUG1	22q12.2	7.1 kb	Upregulated	• Oncogenic • Promotes cell proliferation and invasion	• Interacts with PRC2 • Sponge for miR-9-5p • Decreases POUF2F1 expression • EZH2 upregulation via miR-144-3p • Inhibition of miR-212-3p	[148–150]

lncRNA	Chr. locus	Transcript length	Expression	Function	Mechanisms	Refs
TUSC7	3q13.31	2 kb	Downregulated	• Tumor suppressive	• Affects proapoptotic proteins expression	[189, 190]
UCA1	19p13	2314 bp	Upregulated	• Oncogenic • Promotes cell proliferation • Inhibits cell death • Promotes invasion and metastasis	• Interacts with CREB, BRG1, miR-216b, hnRNP1 • Involvement in PTEN/Akt/Bax/Bcl-2 pathway • Involvement in miR-216b/FGFR1/ERK pathway	[157–161]
ZEB-AS1	2.6 kb	10p11.22	Upregulated	• Oncogenic • Promotes cell proliferation, invasion, and metastasis	• Epigenetic regulation of ZEB1 transcription • Sponge for miR-200s	[169, 170]

Table 1.
Expression, function, and mechanisms of lncRNAs in osteosarcoma.

H19 antisense RNA (91H) has a transcript length of 2.3 kb and is transcribed from the H19/IGF2 genomic imprinted cluster, and its gene is located on chromosome 11p15.5 [93]. It is involved in insulin-like growth factor 2 (IGF2) transcriptional regulation [94, 95]. It has also been observed that the IGF2 and H19 genes are imprinted in the majority of normal human tissues and IGF2 transcriptional repression is regulated through CTCF binding to the H19 imprinting control region [96]. On the other hand, imprinting is lost in various tumor types. Osteosarcoma specimens show maintenance or loss of IGF2/H19 imprinting depending on allele-specific differential methylation of the CTCF-binding regulatory site upstream of H19 gene [97]. Loss of imprinting of IGF2 or H19 in osteosarcoma is mutually exclusive [97]. H19 antisense RNA expression has been found to be elevated in osteosarcoma clinical specimens and osteosarcoma cell line and was correlated with advanced clinical stage. It was considered an independent prognostic factor for overall survival in treated osteosarcoma patients [98]. Moreover, H19 antisense RNA knockdown led to cell death promotion and inhibition of osteosarcoma proliferation, the mechanism of which needs to be elucidated [98].

Antidifferentiation noncoding RNA (ANCR), also called DANCR, is a lncRNA that has been found to suppress osteoblastogenesis through inhibition of Runx2 expression. ANCR interacts with the enhancer of zeste homolog 2 (EZH2). This interaction leads to H3K27me3 catalysis in Runx2 promoter resulting in inhibition of Runx2 expression and suppression of osteogenic differentiation [99]. ANCR also controls the cell cycle progression of osteosarcoma cells through regulation of expression levels of p21, CDK2, and CDK4 and other cell cycle-related proteins as well [100, 101].

Breast cancer antiestrogen resistance 4 (BCAR4) is another lncRNA that has been found to be involved in antiestrogen resistance in breast cancer cell lines [102, 103]. It also promotes cell growth and proliferation as well as invasion and metastasis in breast cancer cell lines, via the noncanonical Hedgehog/GLI2 pathway [75, 98]. In osteosarcoma, BCAR4 exerts its oncogenic action by activating GLI2-dependent gene transcription via direct promoter binding [104]. Upregulation of BCAR4 has been observed in osteosarcoma pathological specimens and is correlated with poor overall survival. Knockdown BCAR4 experiments have shown that suppression of BCAR4 inhibits proliferation and migration in vitro and in vivo through GLI2 target genes [105].

Fibroblast growth factor receptor 3 antisense transcript 1 (FGFR3-AS1), previously known as lncRNA-BX537709, is complimentary to FGFR3 in an antisense direction and increases the mRNA stability and expression of FGFR3 through antisense pairing with the FGFR3 3′UTR [106]. FGFR3-AS1 is upregulated in osteosarcoma along with FGFR3 and is correlated with poor clinical outcome. Knockdown FGFR3-AS1 experiments in osteosarcoma cell lines have demonstrated that suppression of FGFR3-AS1 function leads to inhibition of cell cycle progression and cell proliferation [107].

HIF-2α promoter upstream transcript (HIF2PUT), also named as TCONS_00004241, is located on chromosome 2p21 [80, 108]. It belongs to the class of promoter upstream transcripts lncRNAs (PROMPTs) which regulate host gene transcription [109–111]. In knockdown experiments, suppression of HIF2PUT led to inhibition of expression of HIF-2α and stemness-related genes such as Oct4, Sox, and CD44, resulting in inhibition of cancer stem-cell properties [112]. In osteosarcoma, HIF-2α mRNA and HIF2PUT expression levels are increased and are correlated with advanced clinical stage and poor disease-free and overall survival [80, 108]. HIF2PUT action in osteosarcoma tumorigenesis needs further elucidation in order to understand better its role in osteosarcoma cell self-renewal and stemness.

HOX transcript antisense RNA (HOTAIR) is a 2337-bp-long lncRNA with high expression levels in osteosarcoma tissue clinical specimens [113]. It is implicated in the pathogenesis of various tumors including hepatocellular carcinoma, lung carcinoma, and breast and ovarian cancers [114–117]. It promotes tumor cell growth and proliferation by inhibiting gene expression through histone H3K27 trimethylation, functioning as a modular scaffold by binding PRC2 through the 5′ domain and LSD1/CoREST/REST complexes through the 3′ domain [118, 119]. This molecular mechanism is implicated in other cancer types but remains to be elucidated in osteosarcoma. Interestingly, a genetic variant of HOTAIR, rs7958904, is associated with decreased risk of osteosarcoma in a two-stage case-control study in Chinese population with 900 osteosarcoma cases and 900 controls [120].

HOXA transcript at the distal tip (HOTTIP) is a lncRNA which is overexpressed in osteosarcoma specimens and is correlated with advanced clinical stage and high metastatic potential [121]. Elevated expression of HOTTIP is associated with increased tumor cell proliferation, migration, and invasion in a variety of malignant tumors [122–125]. It exerts its action through regulation of (i) EMT-related molecules such as E-cadherin, Snail1, Slug, etc., (ii) RNA-binding proteins, and (iii) HOXA genes such as HOXA13 [126, 127]. HOTTIP knockdown inhibits cell proliferation, migration, and invasion in osteosarcoma cell lines [42, 128].

Highly upregulated in liver cancer lncRNA (HULC) was initially identified to be upregulated in human hepatocellular carcinoma which has an oncogenic function. Its gene is located on chromosomal locus 6p24.3, has a transcript length of 500 bp, and associates with ribosomes [129, 130]. HULC acts as a sponge for different miRNAs, such as miR200a-3p, miR-9, and miR107, by reducing their expression [131, 132]. It promotes tumor cell growth, invasion, and angiogenesis in hepatocellular and colorectal carcinoma cell lines [133, 134]. HULC is overexpressed in osteosarcoma cell lines and tissue specimens, and its overexpression is correlated with advanced clinical stage and poor overall survival in osteosarcoma patients. HULC inhibition reduces cell proliferation and invasion in osteosarcoma cell lines [135, 136].

Metastasis-associated lung adenocarcinoma transcript 1 (MALAT-1), also called noncoding nuclear-enriched abundant transcrip. 2 (NEAT-2), has a 8.7-kb transcript, and its chromosomal locus is on 11q13 [137]. It is a nuclear lncRNA, initially found to be upregulated in non-small cell lung adenocarcinoma [137, 138]. MALAT-1 functions as a competitive endogenous RNA (ceRNA) by binding to different miRNAs that regulate the transcription of genes such as cell division cycle 2 (cdc2) through miR-1 in breast carcinoma cells [139], Slug through miR-204 in lung adenocarcinoma [140] and metalloproteinase-14 (MMP14), and Snail through miR-22 in melanoma [141]. MALAT-1 is highly expressed in osteosarcoma tissue samples and is correlated with metastatic dissemination and advanced clinical stage [142, 143]. MALAT-1 acts through the PI3K/Akt pathway to promote osteosarcoma cell proliferation, migration, invasion, and pulmonary metastasis [87]. Furthermore, MALAT-1 inhibition suppressed osteosarcoma cell proliferation and metastasis via the PI3K/Akt and RhoA/ROCK signaling pathway by decreasing the expression levels of proliferating cell nuclear antigen (PCNA), Act and phosphorylated PI3Kp85α, as well as MMP-9 metalloproteinase, as mentioned in the signal transduction section [87, 88]. In addition, MALAT-1 may contribute to osteosarcoma tumorigenesis and progression by competing miR376A and promotes TGFα upregulation [144]. MALAT-1 downregulation is also involved in Myc-6 osteosarcoma suppressor activity in MG63 osteosarcoma cell line [145].

Taurine upregulated gene 1 (TUG1) is a 7.1-kb lncRNA, and its gene is located on chromosomal locus 22q12.2 [146]. It seems to be induced by p53, interacts with polycomb repressive complex 2 (PRC2), and suppresses specific genes involved in the G0/G1 cell cycle arrest, facilitating osteosarcoma tumorigenesis [147]. In this context, TUG1 acts as a sponge for miR-9-5p and decreases the expression of POU class 2 homeobox 1 (POUF2F1) supporting the presence of a competitive miR-lncRNA regulatory network [148]. It also promotes osteosarcoma tumorigenesis through EZH2 upregulation via miR-144-3p [149] . Additionally, TUG1 knockdown represses the activation of Wnt/β-catenin pathway, which is reversed by EZH2 upregulation [149]. TUG1 is also involved in osteosarcoma cell proliferation and invasion through inhibition of miR-212-3p [150]. Interestingly, osteosarcoma tissue clinical samples exhibit high expression levels of TUG1, and impairment of TUG1 expression in osteosarcoma cell line U2OS inhibits cell proliferation and promotes cell death [151]. TUG1 is overexpressed in osteosarcoma tissue specimens, and its overexpression is associated with unfavorable prognosis [152].

Urothelial carcinoma associated 1 (UCA1) is a 2314-bp lncRNA located on chromosome 19 and initially identified in bladder carcinoma [153]. It is upregulated in many different tumor types including osteosarcoma, and its overexpression is correlated with high tumor grade, distant metastatic dissemination, advanced clinical stage, and poor clinical outcome [154–156]. Overexpression of UCA1 promotes cancer cell proliferation through interactions with CREB, BRG1, miR-216b, or hnRNP1 [158–161]. On the other hand, UCA1 overexpression inhibits cell death through Akt/Bax/Bcl-2 signaling pathway and promotes migration, invasion, and metastasis via the miR-216b/FGFR1/ERK signal transduction pathway [157–160]. UCA1 upregulation has also been found to be implicated in increased drug resistance through SPRK1, Wnt6, and Wnt signaling pathways [162–164]. UCA1 knockdown experiments in osteosarcoma cell lines have shown that suppression of UCA1 function leads to promotion of cell death and inhibition of cell cycle progression, cell proliferation, cell migration, and invasion, whereas UCA1 upregulation displays opposite effects [160, 165].

Other lncRNAs that play important role in osteosarcoma cell proliferation and display oncogenic properties are:

Modified frailty index 2 (MFI2) is implicated in osteosarcoma development and proliferation by enhancing forkhead box P4 (FOXP4) expression [166].

Small nucleolar RNA host gene 12 (SNHG12) acts by increasing expression of angiomotin gene in human osteosarcoma cell lines and through this action regulates cell proliferation [167]. SNHG12 is also involved in the promotion of osteosarcomagenesis and metastasis through upregulation of Notch2, acting as a sponge for miR-195-p2 in 143B and U2OS osteosarcoma cells [168].

ZEB1 Antisense 1 (ZEB1-AS1) is upregulated in osteosarcoma and promotes osteosarcoma cell proliferation via epigenetic regulation of ZEB1 transcription [169]. ZEB1-AS1 also acts as a sponge for miR-200s and through this action reverses the ZEB1 inhibition caused by miR-200s [170].

3.2 Tumor suppression lncRNAs

Another lncRNA category that plays a significant role in osteosarcoma tumorigenesis includes lncRNAs with tumor suppressive properties such as Loc285194, MEG3, and TUSC7. These lncRNAs are summarized in **Table 1** along with their function and mechanisms.

Loc285194, also named **LSAMP antisense RNA3**, is a 2105-bp lncRNA encoded on chromosomal locus 3q13.31, also called as osteo3q13.31, a locus with frequent copy number alterations and loss of heterozygocity in osteosarcoma [171, 172]. Loc285194 is downregulated in osteosarcoma cell lines and tissue specimens. Loc285194 loss leads to increased osteoblast proliferation through regulation of cell cycle and cell death-related transcripts. It is also implicated in the regulation of VEGF1 transcript [171]. Studies on HCT-116 colon cancer cell line have shown that Loc285194 transcription is regulated by p53 [173, 174] and acts as a tumor suppressor by direct repression of miR-211 in a reciprocal negative feedback loop [175]. This mechanism has not yet been established in osteosarcoma cell lines.

Maternally expressed gene 3 (MEG3) is a lncRNA transcribed by an imprinted gene located on the chromosome 14q32.3 DLK1-MEG3 locus [176]. Reduced or loss of MEG3 expression has been found in many different tumor types such as non-small lung cancer, gastric cancer, colorectal cancer and bladder cancer [177]. The underlying mechanism is through epigenetic promoter or intergenic hypermethylation [178]. Induced expression of MEG3 in different cancer cell lines leads to inhibition of cell proliferation, suppression of migration and invasion, and promotion of apoptosis as well [179–182]. MEG3 overexpression also reduced the expression level of miR21-5p in cervical cancer cells [183], increased the levels of p53, and stimulated the transcription of p53-dependent genes such as MDM2 [184] It is also implicated in the Wnt/β-catenin signaling pathway through regulation of p53, β-catenin, and survivin [185, 186]. Osteosarcoma tissue samples display reduced MEG3 expression levels, and its low expression is associated with distant metastatic dissemination [187, 188]. Further studies are needed to confirm the role of MEG3 in osteosarcoma pathogenesis.

Tumor Suppressor Candidate 7 (TUSC7) is a lncRNA which is downregulated in osteosarcoma cell lines resulting in cell proliferation promotion and increased colony formation in vitro. Decreased expression levels in osteosarcoma tissue specimens are associated with poor survival in osteosarcoma patients. TUSC7 silencing in HOS and MG63 osteosarcoma cells affects the expression of proapoptotic proteins resulting in decreased levels, but with no effect on cell cycle regulation. Moreover MG63 xenografts in nude mice showed tumor growth in vivo after TUSC7 silencing [189, 190].

4. LncRNAs and cell death in osteosarcoma

It is well known that tumor cells enhance their viability by inhibiting apoptosis and anoikis and can survive and metastasize in distant body sites and diverse microenvironments. By inhibiting or reducing the activity of cell death machinery, tumors become resistant to various therapeutic interventions and progress to advanced clinical stages [191–194]. Recent studies have demonstrated the involvement of lncRNAs in osteosarcoma cell death and make them putative therapeutic targets for more efficient osteosarcoma treatment [195, 196].

Reduced **91H** lncRNA expression levels promote osteosarcoma apoptosis via upregulation of miR-141. Overexpression of miR-141 in hFOB1.19 cells leads to osteosarcoma cell apoptosis through the suppression of H19 and miR-675 expression resulting in reduced Bcl-2/Bax ratio and caspase-3 expression [197]. Moreover, knockdown of H19 lncRNA leads to cell death promotion and inhibition of osteosarcoma proliferation.

Inhibition of **BRAF-activated noncoding RNA (BANCR)** lncRNA suppresses MG63 osteosarcoma cell proliferation and invasion in vitro and promotes cell death as well [198].

Metastasis-associated lung adenocarcinoma transcript 1 (MALAT1) lncRNA affects the apoptotic osteosarcoma cell machinery through the RhoA/ROCK signal transduction pathway [88]. MALAT1also regulates osteosarcoma cell proliferation and apoptosis through upregulation of histone deacetylase 4 (HDAC4) by decoying miR-140-5p [199].

Overexpression of **MF12** lncRNA suppresses osteosarcoma cell apoptosis through FOXP4 transcription regulation. Additionally, MF12 knockdown in MG-63 and Saos-2 osteosarcoma cell lines induces apoptosis and reduces cell growth, migration and invasion. [166].

Taurine upregulated gene 1 (TUG1) lncRNA overexpression promotes osteosarcoma tumorigenesis by suppressing specific genes involved in the G0/G1 cell cycle arrest [147]. In this context, TUG1 acts as a sponge for miR-9-5p and decreases the expression of POU class 2 homeobox 1 (POUF2F1) [148]. Suppression of TUG1 has been demonstrated that inhibits cell proliferation and significantly promotes osteosarcoma apoptosis [151].

Silencing of tumor suppressor lncRNA **TUSC7** in HOS and MG63 osteosarcoma cells reduces the expression levels of proapoptotic proteins and results in apoptotic cell reduction [189, 190].

Further studies are needed to explore the role and the precise mechanisms of these lncRNAs in osteosarcoma cell death in an attempt to modulate their action for therapeutic reasons.

5. LncRNAs and invasion/metastasis in osteosarcoma

Despite the introduction of modern treatment approaches by applying multimodality therapies in osteosarcoma patients and the improvement in disease-free survival, the overall long-term survival remains relatively low. In patients with localized disease, the 5-year relapse-free survival is around 75–80% for the good chemoresponders, compared with 45–55% for the poor chemoresponders, in the adjuvant setting and after surgical removal of the bone tumor. The rest of the patients will display mainly pulmonary metastasis by relapsing within the first 5 years, probably because of the presence of undetectable metastatic disease at the time of the initial diagnosis. Approximately, 20–25% of newly diagnosed osteosarcoma patients are presenting with metastatic disease at the initial diagnosis. These patients have an unfavorable prognosis with overall survival rates around 10–30%. It is obvious that the main cause of the high mortality seen in those patients is the development of metastasis, mainly in the lungs [12–18]. Thus, it is important, in order to improve the outcome of patients with metastatic disease, to get insight into the underlying mechanism of osteosarcoma metastasis and develop new therapeutic agents against the metastasis regulatory pathways.

The metastatic process may occur through three main pathways in general: (1) direct invasion of adjacent organs or seeding of body cavities, (2) lymphatic spread, and (3) hematogenous spread. The latter is the main pathway of osteosarcoma metastatic dissemination. A major role in the metastatic cascade plays the phenomenon of epithelial to mesenchymal transition (EMT) whereby epithelial cells lose their epithelial features and acquire mesenchymal cells traits which allow them to invade adjacent tissues and display migratory properties. The metastatic cascade is a multistep complex process and can be divided in the following phases: (1) invasion of the extracellular matrix (ECM) and degradation of ECM proteins through the activity of matrix metalloproteinases (MMPs), (2) intravasation, (3) resistance to anoikis and survival in the peripheral blood, (4) extravasation, and (5) seeding of a distant body site by clones of neoplastic cells with high metastatic potential [192, 200, 201]. A number of studies have shown the involvement of lncRNAs in the metastatic progression of osteosarcoma through modulation of metalloproteinase expression, especially MMP-2 and MMP-9 [202, 203].

Breast cancer antiestrogen resistance 4 (BCAR4) is a lncRNA whose expression has been found to be increased in osteosarcoma tissue specimen in patients with lung metastasis [204]. It acts through transcriptional activation of GLI2-dependent genes via direct promoter binding. Suppression of BCAR4 leads to inhibition of proliferation and migration of osteosarcoma cells in vitro and in vivo through GLI2 target genes [104, 205].

Differentiation antagonizing non-protein coding RNA (DANCR), also named ANCR, is a lncRNA that has been found to be overexpressed in osteosarcoma tissue specimens and in osteosarcoma cell lines. It is involved in osteosarcoma cell proliferation and metastasis through Rho-associated coiled-coil-containing protein kinase 1 (ROCK1) mediation via decoying both miR-335-5p and miR-1972 microRNAs. In this context DANCR acts as a metastasis-promoting lncRNA by playing the role of a competing endogenous RNA (ceRNA) [206].

HOX transcript antisense RNA (HOTAIR) is highly expressed in osteosarcoma and is correlated with distant metastasis and advanced clinical stages. It promotes osteosarcoma invasion through upregulation of metalloproteinases MMP-2 and MMP-9 [207].

Highly up-regulated in liver cancer lncRNA (HULC) acts as a sponge for different miRNAs, such as miR200a-2p, miR-9, and miR107, by reducing their expression [131, 132]. HULC is overexpressed in osteosarcoma cell lines and tissue specimens, and its overexpression is correlated with distant metastasis, advanced clinical stage, and poor overall survival in osteosarcoma patients [135]. It promotes tumor cell growth, invasion, and angiogenesis in different cell lines, and its inhibition reduces cell proliferation and invasion in osteosarcoma cell lines [136].

Long noncoding RNA activated by transforming growth factor-β (lncRNA-ATB) is a novel lncRNA which is activated by the TGF-β and plays a crucial role in many cancers [208]. EMT, and thus invasiveness, can be enhanced by the involvement of the lncRNA-ATB, which acts by interfering the action of miR-200s, a microRNA that suppresses ZEB1 and ZEB2 action [209]. LncRNA-ATB expression levels are high in hepatocellular carcinoma as compared to normal liver samples and are correlated with vascular invasion [210]. Moreover, orthotopic mice injected by hepatocellular carcinoma cells overexpressing lncRNA-ATB developed distant metastasis [211]. LncRNA-ATB promotes osteosarcoma cell proliferation, migration and invasion by inhibiting miR-200s and upregulating the ZEB1 and ZEB2 miR-200s target genes. LncRNA-ATB is also overexpressed in osteosarcoma tissue samples and cell lines and positively correlated with advanced clinical stage, metastasis, and recurrence [212]. The role of lncRNA-ATB in osteosarcoma metastasis is not yet well established, and more studies need to be done in order to elucidate its involvement.

Metastasis-associated lung adenocarcinoma transcript 1 (MALAT-1) facilitates osteosarcoma invasion and metastasis by suppressing the microRNA 376A (miR376A) and promoting TGFα upregulation [144]. MALAT-1 also acts through the PI3K/Akt pathway to promote osteosarcoma cell proliferation, migration, invasion, and pulmonary metastasis. Furthermore, MALAT-1 knockdown or siRNA interference experiments, carried out by Dong et al. and Cai et al., respectively, showed that MALAT1 inhibition suppressed osteosarcoma cell proliferation and metastasis via the PI3K/Akt and RhoA/ROCK signaling pathways by modulating the expression of MMP-9 metalloproteinase [85, 87, 88]. MALAT-1 is highly expressed in osteosarcoma tissue samples and is correlated with metastatic dissemination and advanced clinical stage [142, 143].

Nuclear factor – κB interacting lncRNA (NKILA) is a 2.5-kb lncRNA that negatively regulates the NF-κB pathway. NF-κB is a transcription factor that mediates inflammatory signal transduction processes [213]. It is constitutively active in various tumor types, and its activity can be modulated by interacting with NKILA (nuclear factor-κB interacting lncRNA). NKILA regulates NF-κB activity via interaction with IκBα, a negative regulator of NF-κB translocation from the cytoplasm to the nucleus, thus preventing the transcriptional activation of NF-κB dependent genes [214]. Loss or low expression of NKILA is correlated with advanced clinical stage and metastatic dissemination in breast cancer patients [215]. The role of NKILA in osteosarcoma metastatic dissemination is not well known and remains to be confirmed.

Osteosarcoma doxorubicin resistance-related up-regulated lncRNA (ODRUL) expression levels have been found to be elevated in osteosarcoma tissue specimens of patients with pulmonary metastasis [216]. ODRUL upregulates MMP2 expression through direct competing interaction with miR-3182 and thus promotes invasion and metastasis [217]. ODRUL knockdown experiments in osteosarcoma cell lines led to inhibition of tumor proliferation and invasion by decreasing matrix metalloproteinase (MMP) expression, showing an important role in osteosarcoma metastatic process [217].

P50-associated COX-2 extragenic RNA (PACER) is another lncRNA that acts by promoting osteosarcoma invasion and metastasis through NF-κB-dependent upregulation of COX-2 gene [89].

Small nuclear RNA host gene 12 (SNHG12) lncRNA has been demonstrated to be implicated in the induction of osteosarcoma cell proliferation and migration through the angiomotin upregulation which in turn controls the expression levels of MMP-2 and MMP-9 [167]. SNHG12 is also involved in the promotion of osteosarcomagenesis and metastasis through upregulation of Notch2, acting as a sponge for miR-195-p2 in 143B and U2OS osteosarcoma cells [168].

Zinc finger E-box binding homeobox 1 Antisense 1 (ZEB1-AS1) has been found to display elevated expression levels in metastatic osteosarcoma and regulate the metastatic process by increasing ZEB1 transcription [169]. ZEB1, in turn, promotes invasion and metastasis by inducing epithelial-mesenchymal transition (EMT). ZEB1-AS1 also acts as a sponge for miR-200s and through this action reverses the ZEB1 inhibition caused by miR-200s [170].

Other lncRNAs that play an important role in osteosarcoma invasion and metastasis are:

LncRNA MF12 that has been shown to promote migration of osteosarcoma cells via FOXP4 upregulation [166]. In addition, overexpression of **urothelial carcinoma associated 1 (UCA1)** and **BRAF-activated noncoding RNA (BANCR)** lncRNAs is correlated with metastasis in distant body sites [165, 198].

All the abovementioned lncRNAs are summarized in **Table 1** along with their function and mechanisms.

Further unraveling the mechanism of osteosarcoma invasiveness and metastatic dissemination and the possible involvement of lncRNAs in this process will provide useful insights to develop new therapeutic targets for the management of metastatic osteosarcoma and improve the long-term survival of patients.

6. LncRNAs as prognostic biomarkers in osteosarcoma

The efficacy of osteosarcoma treatment and the accurate prognosis of the clinical outcome depend on clinical, histopathological, and molecular factors, and therefore, it is important to identify and incorporate prognostic factors into a holistic therapeutic strategy. Age, gender, anatomic location, tumor size, and a variety of biological molecules have been used and proposed as a tool to predict the treatment responsiveness and the clinical outcome/prognosis. Recent studies have indicated that lncRNAs may be of clinical value and may be used as prognostic biomarkers in osteosarcoma [106, 128, 218].

Upregulation of **fibroblast growth factor receptor 3 antisense transcript 1 (FGFR3-AS1)** lncRNA is correlated with advanced Enneking surgical stage, large tumor size, and poor clinical outcome and survival [107]. Based on these observations, its expression levels could serve as a prognostic factor.

Interestingly, in a two-stage case-control study in Chinese population performed by Zhou et al., they found that a genetic variant of **HOTAIR,** rs7958904 the CC genotype, was associated with decreased risk of osteosarcoma compared with the G allele (OR, 0.77; 95% CI, 0.67–0.90; $P = 6.77 \times 10^{-4}$). About 900 osteosarcoma patients and 900 control subjects have been evaluated, and the findings suggested that HOTAIR rs7958904 CC genotype patients had significant lower HOTAIR expression levels compared to other genotype patients, as well as lower osteosarcoma risk. Therefore HOTAIR can be used as a prognostic factor for osteosarcoma risk assessment [120].

HOXA transcript at the distal tip (HOTTIP) lncRNA overexpression in osteosarcoma human tissue specimens is associated with distant metastasis, advanced clinical stage, and unfavorable prognosis. Elevated HOTTIP expression levels have been demonstrated to correlate with poor overall survival and to be an independent prognostic factor [121].

Highly upregulated in liver cancer (HULC) lncRNA is overexpressed in osteosarcoma cell lines and tissue specimens, and its overexpression is correlated with advanced clinical stage and poor overall survival in osteosarcoma patients [135, 136]. HULC acts as a sponge for different miRNAs, such as miR200a-2p, miR-9, and miR107, by reducing their expression, and leads to increased cell proliferation, cell migration, and invasion in osteosarcoma cell lines [131, 132, 134, 205]. Inactivation of HULC via knockdown experiments and/or upregulation of miR-122 via transfection of osteosarcoma cell lines results in inactivation of PI3K/Act, Notch, and Jak/Stat pathways leading in reduced proliferation, migration, and invasion [219]. Therefore, HULC could be used as a prognostic factor for osteosarcoma patients as high expression levels are positively correlated with distant metastasis and advanced clinical stage.

Activated by transforming growth factor beta (lncRNA-ATB) displays high expression levels in osteosarcoma cell lines and tissues. Patients with osteosarcoma have elevated serum expression levels of lncRNA-ATB, and this overexpression is correlated with local recurrence, distant metastasis, and advanced clinical stage [208, 212]. Thus, lncRNA-ATB could be used as a prognostic and recurrence monitoring factor for osteosarcoma patients.

Maternally expressed gene 3 (MEG3) lncRNA expression levels are decreased in osteosarcoma tissues compared with adjacent normal tissues and are associated with distant metastasis, advanced clinical stage, and poor overall survival [177, 220]. Its expression is regulated by lncRNA Ewing sarcoma associated transcript 1 (EWSAT1) and downregulation of MEG3 in the presence of EWSAT1 induces osteosarcoma cell proliferation, invasion, and metastasis [221]. Therefore, high levels of MEG3 could be an indicator of favorable prognosis in osteosarcoma patients.

Taurine upregulated gene 1 (TUG1) lncRNA has been found to be overexpressed in osteosarcoma human samples compared with normal matched tissues ($P < 0.01$), and expression levels were associated with tumor size, postoperative chemotherapy responsiveness and Enneking surgical stage [152]. Moreover, TUG1 high expression levels were significantly correlated with unfavorable prognosis and were an independent prognostic factor for disease-free survival ($HR = 1.81$; 95% CI = 1.01–3.54; $P = 0.037$) and long-term overall survival ($HR = 2.78$; 95% CI = 1.29–6.00; $P = 0.009$). Interestingly, TUG1 elevated plasma levels are associated with disease progression or relapse [152]. Thus, TUG1 might be used as a prognostic and monitoring biomarker for osteosarcoma patients.

lncRNA	Expression in osteosarcoma	Clinical value	Role in drug resistance or sensitivity	Mechanism of drug resistance or sensitivity	Therapeutic target	Agent targeting lncRNA	Refs
BCAR4	Upregulated	Prognostic, therapeutic			Yes	Antagonist	[105, 204, 205]
BANCR	Upregulated	Prognostic, predictive	Adriamycin resistance	—			[198]
CASC2	Downregulated	Prognostic, therapeutic			Yes	Agonist-mimic	[242]
FENDRR	Downregulated	Predictive, therapeutic	Doxorubicin resistance	• Upregulated acts as a suppressor of doxorubicin resistance by inhibiting ABCB1 and ABCC1 expression	Yes	Agonist-mimic	[229]
FGFR3-AS1	Upregulated	Prognostic					[107]
FOXC2-AS1	Upregulated	Prognostic, predictive	Doxorubicin resistance	Induces ABCB1 gene expression			[230]
GAS5	Downregulated	Prognostic, therapeutic			Yes	Agonist-mimic	[243, 244]
HOTAIR	Upregulated	Prognostic, risk assessment					[120, 207]
HOTTIP	Upregulated	Prognostic, predictive	Cisplatin resistance	• Activates Wnt/β-catenin pathway			[231]
HULC	Upregulated	Prognostic					[135, 136]
LINC00161	Upregulated	Predictive	Cisplatin sensitivity	• Promotes apoptosis • Increases IFIT2 expression • Sponge for miR-645			[232]
LncRNA-ATB	Upregulated	Prognostic, monitoring marker					[212]
LUCAT1	Upregulated	Predictive	Methotrexate resistance	• Interacts with ABCB1 through miR-200c • Regulates miR-200c expression			[235]

DOI: http://dx.doi.org/10.5772/intechopen.83847

lncRNA	Expression in osteosarcoma	Clinical value	Role in drug resistance or sensitivity	Mechanism of drug resistance or sensitivity	Therapeutic target	Agent targeting lncRNA	Refs
MALAT-1	Upregulated	Prognostic, therapeutic			Yes	Antagonist	[142, 143, 246]
MEG3	Downregulated	Prognostic					[188, 220]
MF12	Upregulated	Prognostic, therapeutic			Yes	Antagonist	[166]
NBAT1	Downregulated	Prognostic, therapeutic			Yes	Agonist-mimic	[248]
NR-036444	Upregulated	Predictive	Doxorubicin resistance	Interacts with ABCB1, HIF1α, and FOXC2			[236]
ODRUL	Upregulated	Prognostic, predictive	Doxorubicin resistance	Induces ABCB1 gene expression			[217, 237]
PANDA	Upregulated	Prognostic, therapeutic	Doxorubicin resistance	• Increased expression after doxorubicin and etoposide treatment • Depletion promotes apoptosis through upregulation of APAF1, BIK, FAS, and LRDD	Yes	Antagonist	[249, 250]
PVT1	Upregulated	Prognostic, therapeutic			Yes	Antagonist	[251, 252]
TP73-AS1	Upregulated	Prognostic, therapeutic			Yes	Antagonist	[253, 254]
TUG1	Upregulated	Prognostic, monitoring marker					[152]
ZEB1-AS1	Upregulated	Prognostic					[169]

Table 2.
Potential clinical value of lncRNAs in osteosarcoma.

Zinc finger E-box binding homeobox 1 antisense 1 (ZEB1-AS1) has been found to display elevated expression levels in metastatic osteosarcoma and regulate the metastatic process by increasing ZEB1 transcription [169, 170]. Overexpression of ZEB1-AS1 is associated with advanced clinical stage, large tumor size, distant metastatic dissemination, and unfavorable progression-free and overall survival [169]. In clinical setting, ZEB1-AS1 could serve as a prognostic marker for osteosarcoma patients.

All the abovementioned lncRNAs are summarized in **Table 2**.

7. LncRNAs as predictive biomarkers and drug resistance in osteosarcoma

A number of research teams have demonstrated the involvement of lncRNAs in chemoresistance and chemosensitivity of different types of cancer [222–227]. In osteosarcoma, chemotherapy plays an important role, but its efficacy is limited by acquired resistance to different chemotherapeutic drugs, mainly cisplatin and doxorubicin [228]. Recent studies have revealed the role of several lncRNAs that are related to osteosarcoma drug resistance such as FENDRR, ENST00000563280, HOTTIP, LINC00161, LUCAT1, NR-036444, and ODRUL [106].

FENDRR is another lncRNA which is significantly downregulated in doxorubicin-resistant osteosarcoma cell lines compared with the doxorubicin-sensitive counterparts (MG63/DXR vs. MG63, KH-OS/DXR vs. KH-OS, and U2-OS/DXR vs. U2-OS). In a microarray study FENDRR displayed a 22-fold decrease of its expression in doxorubicin-resistant MG63/DXR cells relative to their parental cell line MG63. It has been demonstrated that it acts as a suppressor of doxorubicin drug resistance by inhibiting ABCB1 and ABCC1 expressions [229].

Another lncRNA related with doxorubicin resistance in osteosarcoma cell lines is **forkhead box protein C2 antisense 1 (FOXC2-AS1)** also known as **ENST00000563280**. FOXC2-AS1 has been found to have elevated expression levels in osteosarcoma tissues and osteosarcoma cell lines resistant to doxorubicin, such as MG-63 and KH-OS. FOXC2-AS1 overexpression is associated with unfavorable clinical outcome and promotion of doxorubicin resistance in cell cultures. FOXC2-AS1 knockdown reversed the doxorubicin resistant phenotype and increased the doxorubicin sensitivity in osteosarcoma cells resistant to doxorubicin [230]. In addition, FOXC2 is overexpressed in osteosarcoma doxorubicin-resistant human tissues and cell lines, such as MG63/DXR and KH-OS/DXR, and its levels show positive correlation with FOXC2-AS1 expression. Both FOXC2-AS1 and FOXC2 are involved in doxorubicin resistance by inducing the expression of ABCB1 multidrug resistance gene [230]. Therefore, FOXC2-AS1 might serve as a predictive factor for doxorubicin sensitivity or resistance in osteosarcoma patients.

HOTTIP lncRNA is overexpressed in osteosarcoma specimens and is correlated with advanced clinical stage and high metastatic potential [121]. In a recent study, Li et al. found that overexpression of HOTTIP confers resistance to cisplatin in osteosarcoma cells in vitro through activation of the Wnt/β-catenin pathway. Moreover, treatment with Wnt/β-catenin inhibitor XAV939 or downregulation of HOTTIP reverses the cisplatin resistance [231]. Thus, HOTTIP expression levels might serve as a predictive biomarker regarding cisplatin resistance in osteosarcoma.

Long intergenic non-protein coding RNA 161 (LINC00161) is a lncRNA located on chromosome 21q21 locus and has been found to be overexpressed in cisplatin-treated osteosarcoma cells facilitating the cisplatin-induced apoptosis. Upregulation of LINC00161 in osteosarcoma cells promotes apoptosis by increasing

IFIT2 expression levels through the impairment of miR-645 action. In this context, LINC00161 acts as a sponge for miR-645, a microRNA that controls IFIT2 transcription [232].

Lung cancer associated transcript 1 (LUCAT1) lncRNA has been found to be overexpressed in osteosarcoma tissue samples and in MG63 and HOX osteosarcoma cell lines resistant to methotrexate, a drug that is used widely in osteosarcoma patients [233–235]. MG63 and HOX, resistant to methotrexate, also overexpress the ATP-binding cassette subfamily B member 1 (ABCB1), a drug resistance-related protein. LUCAT1 interacts with ABCB1 through miR-200c binding to the 3′UTR of ABCB1. Moreover, miR-200c expression is regulated in a LUCAT1-dependent manner. In addition, LUCAT1 knockdown experiments resulted in decreased expression levels of drug resistance-related genes MDR1, MRP5, and LRP1 in methotrexate-treated osteosarcoma cell lines and led to reduced osteosarcoma cell invasiveness [235]. Therefore, LUCAT1 expression levels might be used as a predictive biomarker providing information regarding methotrexate resistance or sensitivity.

NR-036444 is another lncRNA involved in an lncRNA-mRNA coexpression network and has been found to interact with doxorubicin-resistance related genes such as ABCB1, HIF1A, and FOXC2 in osteosarcoma cells and thus could serve as a predictive biomarker for chemoresistance [236].

Osteosarcoma doxorubicin resistance-related up-regulated lncRNA (ODRUL) has been initially found to be highly upregulated in the human osteosarcoma doxorubicin-resistant cell line MG63/DXR. Moreover ODRUL expression is elevated in human tissue osteosarcoma specimens from patients with poor response to doxorubicin therapy and lung metastasis. It has also been found that doxorubicin-sensitive osteosarcoma cell lines have reduced ODRUL expression levels. Additionally, ODRUL knockdown experiments in osteosarcoma cell lines led to inhibition of tumor proliferation and invasion and partly reversed the doxorubicin resistant phenotype through suppression of the multidrug resistance ABCB1 (ATP-binding cassette, subfamily B, member 1) gene [217, 237].

All the abovementioned lncRNAs are summarized in **Table 2**.

Further studies are needed to elucidate the role of lncRNAs in osteosarcoma drug resistance and exploit their potential as predictive biomarkers and candidates to develop novel therapeutic approaches in order to reverse the osteosarcoma resistance to chemotherapy.

8. LncRNAs as therapeutic targets in osteosarcoma

Treating osteosarcoma is a challenge in the practice of oncology. The main therapeutic approach is surgical removal of the tumor following by the application of chemotherapeutic agents such as doxorubicin, cisplatin, methotrexate in combination with leucovorin (folinic acid), and ifosfamide [13, 233]. This multimodal osteosarcoma management increased the progression-free survival rates from 10 to 20% up to 60% in recent years. Despite the relatively good cure rates of patients with localized tumor, unfortunately a percentage of 20–25% of newly diagnosed osteosarcoma patients are presenting with metastatic disease at the time of initial diagnosis. These patients have an unfavorable prognosis with overall survival rates around 10–30% [12–18]. In addition many patients develop resistance to available chemotherapeutic modalities and subsequently metastatic dissemination with unfavorable clinical outcome [228]. In recent years there are great efforts to exploit the molecular mechanisms of the metastatic process and drug resistance of osteosarcoma in order to develop novel therapeutic agents targeting biomolecules involved in these processes. Such biomolecules, among others, are the lncRNAs which play important roles in the pathogenesis and progression of osteosarcoma [238–240].

Breast cancer antiestrogen resistance 4 (BCAR4) is another lncRNA that promotes cell growth and proliferation as well as invasion and metastasis in breast cancer cell lines cultures, via the noncanonical Hedgehog/GLI2 pathway [103, 104]. In osteosarcoma, BCAR4 exerts its oncogenic action by activating GLI2-dependent gene transcription via direct promoter binding [104]. Upregulation of BCAR4 has been observed in osteosarcoma pathological specimens and is correlated with advanced clinical stage, lung metastasis, and poor overall survival [105]. Knock-down BCAR4 experiments have shown that suppression of BCAR4 leads to inhibition of cell proliferation and migration in vitro and in vivo through downregulation of GLI2 target genes, such as IL-6, TGF-beta, RPS3, and MUC5AC [104]. Thus BCAR4 could be used as a target in osteosarcoma therapeutic management [205].

Cancer susceptibility candidate 2 (CASC2) was first discovered in patients with endometrial carcinoma as a potential tumor suppressor [241]. It is also significantly downregulated in osteosarcoma human specimens and various osteosarcoma cell lines such as MG-63, Saos-2, U2OS, and SOSP-9607, and its low expression levels correlate with poor survival and advanced clinical stage [241]. Interestingly, overexpression of CASC2 results in inhibition of osteosarcoma cell proliferation, colony formation, and invasion in vitro. Ectopic expression of CASC2 suppresses miR-181a expression and leads to upregulation of miR-181a target genes such as RASSF6, PTEN, and ATM in osteosarcoma cell lines. RASSF6 has been observed to positively correlate with CASC2 expression levels, and low RASSF6 levels have been found in osteosarcoma. In addition, in vivo implantation studies using pcDNA-CASC2 resulted in reduced tumor growth, while experiments using short interfering CASC2 exhibited enhanced tumor growth [242]. Consequently, CASC2 mimics might be of clinical value in osteosarcoma treatment in order to reduce tumor growth and slow down adverse clinical progression.

LncRNA growth arrest-specific 5 (GAS5) functions as an oncosuppressor lncRNA by repressing osteosarcoma cell proliferation and migration through sponging of miR-203a. In addition, silencing of lncRNA GAS5 significantly promotes osteosarcoma cell growth, migration, and invasion through upregulation of Cyclin D1, Cyclin B1, CDK1, and CDK4 expressions. Moreover, suppression of miR-203a leads to the reversion of GAS5 silencing effects [243]. GAS5 also functions as a ceRNA by binding to miR-221 resulting in the suppression of epithelial-mesenchymal transition and arrest of cell growth in osteosarcoma cell lines through regulation of the miR-221/ARHI axis [244]. Thus, GAS5 mimics could be used to slow down or suppress the osteosarcoma metastatic process.

Metastasis-associated lung adenocarcinoma transcript 1 (MALAT1) is an oncogenic lncRNA that is overexpressed in various osteosarcoma cell lines such as U2OS, Saos-2, and HOS and in human osteosarcoma tissue samples as well. Its overexpression is highly related to the metastatic potential of the tumor [142, 143]. MALAT1 acts through the PI3K/Akt and the RhoA/ROCK signaling pathway to promote osteosarcoma cell proliferation, migration, invasion, and pulmonary metastasis [87]. Downregulation of MALAT1 leads to reduced expression levels of RhoA and ROCK1 and 2 in osteosarcoma cell lines [87, 88]. Moreover, MALAT1 knockdown induces cell cycle arrest at the G0/G1 to S phase leading to reduced cell proliferation and invasion and enhanced apoptosis in HOS and U2OS cell lines. In addition, MALAT1 knockdown affects negatively the ability of osteosarcoma cells to form new blood circulatory networks in three-dimensional cell cultures [88, 245]. In addition, MALAT1 knockdown inactivates the Rac1/JNK signal transduction pathway through activation of miR-509 and downregulation of high mobility group protein B1 (HMGB1) [246, 247]. It is obvious that inactivation of MALAT1 results in inhibition of osteosarcoma cell proliferation and invasion and induces the apoptotic machinery. Therefore, MALAT1 might be used as specific therapeutic target to inhibit osteosarcoma progression.

MF12 is another lncRNA that is overexpressed in osteosarcoma human tissue samples and is associated with cell proliferation, migration, and invasion in osteosarcoma cell lines MG63 and Saos-2. It promotes osteosarcoma cell growth and enhances invasiveness through regulation of FOXP4 [166]. In this context, targeting MF12 could reduce osteosarcoma growth and clinical progression.

Neuroblastoma-associated transcript 1 (NBAT1) has been found to be downregulated in osteosarcoma human samples and various osteosarcoma cell lines such as MG-63, KHOA, U2OS, LM7, and 143b [248]. Clinically, low expression levels of NBAT1 are associated with osteosarcoma metastatic dissemination and unfavorable prognosis. NBAT1 knockdown or silencing leads to enhanced osteosarcoma tumor growth, cell proliferation, migration and invasion in vitro. Induction of NBAT1, in order to be overexpressed in vitro, results in the opposite effects. It has also been demonstrated that NBAT1 positively regulates the transcription of PTEN, PDCD4 and RECK, which act as tumor suppressor, and cell death and metastasis suppressor genes, respectively, through miR-21 inactivation. Overexpression of miR-21 leads to the opposite effect [248]. Thus, NBAT1 mimics might be used to reduce osteosarcoma growth and metastatic ability.

p21-associated ncRNA DNA damage activated (PANDA) is a lncRNA which is overexpressed in osteosarcoma tissue specimens and osteosarcoma cell lines [249]. Its expression is induced up to 40-fold by DNA damage related to doxorubicin and etoposide treatment and is positively regulated by p53. PANDA is involved in positive regulation of the osteosarcoma cell cycle through p18 associated transcriptional repression. Moreover, PANDA silencing results in cell cycle arrest in G1/S transition through upregulation of cyclin-dependent kinase inhibitor p18 in U2OS osteosarcoma cell line. Depletion of PANDA leads to cell death of doxorubicin treated cells through upregulation of apoptotic activators APAF1, BIK, FAS, and LRDD [249, 250]. Taken together, these findings imply that inhibition of PANDA might serve as a therapeutic intervention to induce cell cycle arrest and apoptosis in osteosarcoma.

PVT1 is another lncRNA that is overexpressed in osteosarcoma cell lines and tissue specimens, and its upregulation is correlated with decreased survival in osteosarcoma patients. PVT1 overexpression is associated with osteosarcoma cell proliferation, migration, and invasion, and silencing of its function via siRNA has the opposite effects and promotes apoptosis and cell cycle arrest as well. Moreover, silencing of PVT1 by siRNA leads to downregulation of BCL2, CCND1, and FASN expressions through miR-195 in osteosarcoma cells [251]. PVT1 is also involved in the Warburg effect in osteosarcoma cells by promoting anaerobic glycolysis and tumor progression through regulation of the miR-497/HK2 axis [252]. Taken together, PVT1 could serve as a target in the therapeutic management of osteosarcoma.

TP73 antisense RNA 1 (TP73-AS1) is a novel oncogenic long noncoding RNA which is significantly overexpressed in osteosarcoma tissue samples and cell lines. Moreover, high expression of TP73-AS1 is correlated with advanced clinical stage, large tumor size, high metastatic potential, and poor overall survival [253]. TP73-AS1 overexpression promotes osteosarcoma cell proliferation, migration, and invasion by acting as a sponge for miR-142 to positively regulate Rac1 function [254]. TP73-AS1 might constitute a potential therapeutic target in the treatment of osteosarcoma.

All the above mentioned lncRNAs are summarized in **Table 2**.

Different methods and approaches could be used to inhibit or mimic the function of lncRNAs for therapeutic purposes, such as small molecule inhibitors, inhibiting micropeptides; RNA interference silencing by small interfering RNAs (siRNAs); or short hairpin RNAs (shRNAs), antisense oligonucleotide targeting; ribozyme, deoxyribozyme, plasmid, or viral vector-based targeting; and gene editing by CRISPR/Cas9 system [255].

In addition, a variety of delivery vehicles or carriers have been developed in an effort to target lncRNAs, such as peptide nucleic acid (PNA), lipid-based nanocarriers, poly(lactic-co-glycolic acid nanoparticles (PLGA), poly(amine-co-ester) tetrapolymers (PACE), and pHlow insertion peptides (pHLIP) [256].

Several preclinical and phaseI/II clinical trials have been initiated by using the abovementioned approaches, such as the use of plasmid BC-819 expressing diphtheria toxin under the control of H19 lncRNA promoter to induce tumor reduction after intratumoral injection in order to treat bladder, ovarian, and pancreatic carcinomas [256]. Modified oligonucleotides which target antisense lncRNAs, also referred as AntagoNATs, have been tested *in vitro* and *in vivo* to modulate lncRNA expression. Administration of antisense oligonucleotides (ASOs) against MALAT1 effectively achieved inhibition of lung cancer tumor growth in mice xenografts [257]. Although ASO therapeutic approaches are promising, major obstacles, such as inadequate intracellular uptake or chemical toxicity, should be considered and taken into account. It should also be noted that although lncRNAs are regulated by *cis* or *trans* mechanisms targeting specific genes, putative effects on global gene expression should be very carefully considered.

9. Conclusions and future perspectives

In this chapter, we reviewed the involvement of lncRNAs in the pathogenesis, metastatic process, and drug resistance of osteosarcoma and summarized in **Tables 1** and 2. We also summarized the possible roles of lncRNAs as prognostic and predictive biomarkers and their putative usefulness as therapeutic targets in osteosarcoma clinical management. However, more studies are needed to further elucidate and confirm the precise molecular mechanisms underlying these effects along with translational research in osteosarcoma metastasis and drug resistance. Translational studies are crucial in understanding if lncRNA modulation is applicable in the clinical setting and beneficial for the patients. Considering the difficulty to get osteosarcoma tissue samples at different stages of disease, it would be useful to detect lncRNA expression levels in body fluids, such as plasma or urine, providing a real-time monitoring of osteosarcoma progression [45, 258].

Studies of structural biology are also needed in order to determine the secondary and tertiary structures of lncRNAs and elucidate the molecular interactions with other biomolecules. Structural studies could provide useful knowledge for designing lncRNA mimics or pharmaceutical agents against them.

Future research should also focus on better understanding the cross-talk between different signaling pathways related to osteosarcoma development and the role of lncRNAs in these molecular interactions.

We anticipate that lncRNA-based diagnostic approaches and therapeutic interventions will be more efficient in treating this debilitating tumor and will offer significant benefit for osteosarcoma patients.

Author details

Christos Valavanis* and Gabriela Stanc
Department of Pathology, Molecular Pathology Unit, "Metaxa Cancer Hospital", Piraeus, Greece

*Address all correspondence to: cvalapath@yahoo.com

References

[1] Messerschmitt PJ, Garcia RM, Abdul-Karim FW, Greenfield EM, Getty PJ. Osteosarcoma. The Journal of the American Academy of Orthopaedic Surgeons. 2009;**17**:515-527

[2] Ottaviani G, Jaffe N. The epidemiology of osteosarcoma. Cancer Treatment and Research. 2009;**152**:3-13. DOI: 10.1007/978-1-4419-0284-9_1

[3] Mirabello L, Troisi RJ, Savage SA. International osteosarcoma incidence patterns in children and adolescents, middle ages and elderly persons. International Journal of Cancer. 2009; **125**:229-234. DOI: 10.1002/ijc.24320

[4] Trihia H, Valavanis C. Histopathology and molecular pathology of bone and extraskeletal osteosarcomas. In: Manish A, editor. Osteosarcoma. Rijeka, Croatia: IntechOpen; 2012. pp. 3-40. DOI: 10.5772/31431

[5] Bousquet M, Noirot C, Accadbled F, Sales de Gauzy J, Castex MP, Brousset P, et al. Whole-exome sequencing in osteosarcoma reveals important heterogeneity of genetic alterations. Annals of Oncology. 2016;**27**:738-744. DOI: 10.1093/annonc/mdw009

[6] Smida J, Baumhoer D, Rosemann M, et al. Genomic alterations and allelic imbalances are strong prognostic predictors in osteosarcoma. Clinical Cancer Research. 2010;**16**(16): 4256-4267. DOI: 10.1158/1078-0432. CCR-10-0284

[7] Stock C, Kager L, Fink FM, Gadner H, Ambros PF. Chromosomal regions involved in the pathogenesis of osteosarcomas. Genes, Chromosomes & Cancer. 2000;**28**:329-336

[8] Atiye J, Wolf M, Kaur S, Monni O, Bohling T, Kivioja A, et al. Gene amplifications in osteosarcoma-CGH microarray analysis. Genes, Chromosomes & Cancer. 2005;**42**: 158-163. DOI: 10.1002/gcc.20120

[9] Liu JJ, Liu S, Wang JG, Zhu W, Hua YQ, Sun W, et al. Telangiectatic osteosarcoma: A review of literature. OncoTargets and Therapy. 2013;**6**: 593-602. DOI: 10.2147/OTT.S41351

[10] Fletcher CDM, Hogendoorn Pancras CW, Mertens F, Bridge J. WHO Classification of Tumours of Soft Tissue and Bone (Medicine). 4th ed. WHO; Lyon, France: IARC Press; 2013. pp. 264-285. ISBN-10: 9283224345

[11] Sathiyamoorthy S, Ali SZ. Osteoblastic osteosarcoma: Cytomorphologic characteristics and differential diagnosis on fine-needle aspiration. Acta Cytologica. 2012;**56**: 481-486

[12] Miller BJ, Cram P, Lynch CF, Buckwalter JA. Risk factors for metastatic disease at presentation with osteosarcoma: An analysis of the SEER database. The Journal of Bone and Joint Surgery. American Volume. 2013;**95** (e89):1-8. DOI: 10.2106/JBJS.L.01189

[13] Bielack S, Carrle D, Casali PG, Group EGW. Osteosarcoma: ESMO clinical recommendations for diagnosis, treatment and follow-up. Annals of Oncology. 2009;**20**:137-139. DOI: 10.1093/annonc/mdp154

[14] Eilber F, Giuliano A, Eckardt J, Patterson K, Moseley S, Goodnight J. Adjuvant chemotherapy for osteosarcoma: A randomized prospective trial. Journal of Clinical Oncology. 1987;**5**:21-26

[15] Allison DC, Carney SC, Ahlmann ER, Hendifar A, Chawla S, Fedenko A, et al. A meta-analysis of osteosarcoma outcomes in the modern medical era. Sarcoma. 2012;**2012**:704872

[16] Meyers PA, Heller G, Healey JH, Huvos A, Applewhite A, Sun M, et al. Osteogenic sarcoma with clinically detectable metastasis at initial presentation. Journal of Clinical Oncology. 1993;**11**:449-453

[17] Kager L, Zoubek A, Pötschger U, Kastner U, Flege S, Kempf-Bielack B, et al. Cooperative German-Austrian-Swiss Osteosarcoma Study Group. Primary metastatic osteosarcoma: Presentation and outcome of patients treated on neoadjuvant Cooperative Osteosarcoma Study Group protocols. Journal of Clinical Oncology. 2003;**21**: 2011-2018. DOI: 10.1200/JCO.2003. 08.132

[18] Daw NC, Billups CA, Rodriguez-Galindo C, McCarville MB, Rao BN, Cain AM, et al. Metastatic osteosarcoma. Cancer. 2006;**106**:403-412

[19] Diamantopoulos MA, Tsiakanikas P, Scorilas A. Non-coding RNAs: The riddle of the transcriptome and their perspectives in cancer. Annals of Translational Medicine. 2018;**6**(12):241. DOI: 10.21037/atm.2018.06.10

[20] Kunej T, Obsteter J, Pogacar Z, Horvat S, Calin GA. The decalog of long non-coding RNA involvement in cancer diagnosis and monitoring. Critical Reviews in Clinical Laboratory Sciences. 2014;**51**(6):344-357. DOI: 10.3109/ 10408363.2014.944299

[21] Crea F, Clermont PL, Parolia A, Wang Y, Helgason CD. The non-coding transcriptome as a dynamic regulator of cancer metastasis. Cancer Metastasis Reviews. 2013;**33**(1):1-16. DOI: 10.1007/ s10555-013-9455-3

[22] Cech TR, Steitz JA. The noncoding RNA revolution—Trashing old rules to forge new ones. Cell. 2014;**157**(1):77-94. DOI: 10.1016/j.cell.2014.03.008

[23] Sandberg K, Samson WK, Ji H. Decoding noncoding RNA: The long and short of it. Circulation Research. 2013; **113**(3):240-241. DOI: 10.1161/ CIRCRESAHA. 113.301865

[24] Kawaguchi T, Tanigawa A, Naganuma T, et al. SWI/SNF chromatin-remodeling complexes function in noncoding RNA-dependent assembly of nuclear bodies. Proceedings of the National Academy of Sciences of the United States of America. 2015; **112**(14):4304-4309. DOI: 10.1073/pnas. 1423819112

[25] Zhu Y, Rowley MJ, Böhmdorfer G, Wierzbicki AT. A SWI/SNF chromatin-remodeling complex acts in noncoding RNA-mediated transcriptional silencing. Molecular Cell. 2013;**49**(2):298-309. DOI: 10.1016/j.molcel.2012.11.011

[26] Tang Y, Wang J, Lian Y, et al. Linking long non-coding RNAs and SWI/SNF complexes to chromatin remodeling in cancer. Molecular Cancer. 2017;**16**(1):42. DOI: 10.1186/s12943-017-0612-0

[27] St Laurent G, Wahlestedt C, Kapranov P. The landscape of long noncoding RNA classification. Trends in Genetics. 2015;**31**(5):239-251. DOI: 10.1016/j.tig.2015.03.007

[28] Ponting CP, Oliver PL, Reik W. Evolution and functions of long noncoding RNAs. Cell. 2009;**136**: 629-641. DOI: 10.1016/j.cell.2009.02.006

[29] Batista PJ, Chang HY. Long noncoding RNAs: Cellular address codes in development and disease. Cell. 2013; **152**(6):1298-1307. DOI: 10.1016/j.cell. 2013.02.012

[30] Wang KC, Chang HY. Molecular mechanisms of long noncoding RNAs. Molecular Cell. 2011;**43**:904-914. DOI: 10.1016/j.molcel.2011.08.018

[31] Ma L, Bajic VB, Zhang Z. On the classification of long non-coding RNAs.

RNA Biology. 2013;**10**(6):925-933. DOI: 10.4161/rna.24604

[32] Gibb EA, Brown CJ, Lam WL. The functional role of long non-coding RNA in human carcinomas. Molecular Cancer. 2011;**10**:38. DOI: 10.1186/1476-4598-10-38

[33] El Khodiry A, Afify M, El Tayebi HM. Behind the curtain of non-coding RNAs; long non-coding RNAs regulating hepatocarcinogenesis. World Journal of Gastroenterology. 2018; **24**(5):549-572. DOI: 10.3748/wjg.v24.i5.549

[34] Ragusa M, Barbagallo C, Statello L, et al. Non-coding landscapes of colorectal cancer. World Journal of Gastroenterology. 2015;**21**(41): 11709-11739. DOI: 10.3748/wjg.v21.i41.11709

[35] Heery R, Finn SP, Cuffe S, Gray SG. Long non-coding RNAs: Key regulators of epithelial-mesenchymal transition, tumour drug resistance and cancer stem cells. Cancers (Basel). 2017;**9**(4):38. DOI: 10.3390/cancers9040038

[36] Cerk S, Schwarzenbacher D, Adiprasito JB, et al. Current status of long non-coding RNAs in human breast cancer. International Journal of Molecular Sciences. 2016;**17**(9):1485. DOI: 10.3390/ijms17091485

[37] Gulìa C, Baldassarra S, Signore F, et al. Role of non-coding RNAs in the etiology of bladder cancer. Genes (Basel). 2017;**8**(11):339. DOI: 10.3390/genes8110339

[38] Silva A, Bullock M, Calin G. The clinical relevance of long non-coding RNAs in cancer. Cancers (Basel). 2015; **7**(4):2169-2182. DOI: 10.3390/cancers7040884

[39] Huarte M. The emerging role of lncRNAs in cancer. Nature Medicine. 2015;**21**(11):1253-1261. DOI: 10.1038/nm.3981

[40] Schmitt AM, Chang HY. Long noncoding RNAs in cancer pathways. Cancer Cell. 2016;**29**(4):452-463. DOI: 10.1016/j.ccell.2016.03.010

[41] Corrà F, Agnoletto C, Minotti L, Baldassari F, Volinia S. The network of non-coding RNAs in cancer drug resistance. Frontiers in Oncology. 2018; **8**:327. DOI: 10.3389/fonc.2018.00327

[42] Chen R, Wang G, Zheng Y, Hua Y, Cai Z. Long non-coding RNAs in osteosarcoma. Oncotarget. 2017;**8**(12): 20462-20475. DOI: 10.18632/oncotarget.14726

[43] Min L, Garbutt C, Tu C, Hornicek F, Duan Z. Potentials of long noncoding RNAs (LncRNAs) in sarcoma: From biomarkers to therapeutic targets. International Journal of Molecular Sciences. 2017;**18**(4):731. DOI: 10.3390/ijms18040731

[44] Yang Z, Li X, Yang Y, He Z, Qu X, Zhang Y. Long noncoding RNAs in the progression, metastasis, and prognosis of osteosarcoma. Cell Death & Disease. 2016;**7**(9):e2389. DOI: 10.1038/cddis.2016.272

[45] Smolle MA, Pichler M. The role of long non-coding RNAs in osteosarcoma. Noncoding RNA. 2018;**4**(1):7. DOI: 10.3390/ncrna4010007

[46] Lin YH, Jewell BE, Gingold J, et al. Osteosarcoma: Molecular pathogenesis and iPSC modeling. Trends in Molecular Medicine. 2017;**23**(8):737-755. DOI: 10.1016/j.molmed.2017.06.004

[47] Morrow JJ, Khanna C. Osteosarcoma genetics and epigenetics: Emerging biology and candidate therapies. Critical Reviews in Oncogenesis. 2015;**20**(3–4):173-197. DOI: 10.1615/CritRevOncog.2015013713

[48] Peng WX, Koirala P, Mo YY. LncRNA-mediated regulation of cell signaling in cancer. Oncogene. 2017; **36**(41):5661-5667. DOI: 10.1038/onc.2017.184

[49] Yao Z, Han L, Chen Y, et al. Hedgehog signalling in the tumourigenesis and metastasis of osteosarcoma, and its potential value in the clinical therapy of osteosarcoma. Cell Death & Disease. 2018;**9**(6):701. DOI: 10.1038/s41419-018-0647-1

[50] Mao X, Su Z, Mookhtiar AK. Long non-coding RNA: A versatile regulator of the nuclear factor-κB signalling circuit. Immunology. 2017;**150**(4): 379-388. DOI: 10.1111/imm.12698

[51] Wang Y, Li YP, Paulson C, et al. Wnt and the Wnt signaling pathway in bone development and disease. Frontiers in Bioscience (Landmark Ed). 2014;**19**:379-407. http://dx.doi.org/10.2741/4214

[52] Boland GM, Perkins G, Hall DJ, Tuan RS. Wnt 3a promotes proliferation and suppresses osteogenic differentiation of adult human mesenchymal stem cells. Journal of Cellular Biochemistry. 2004;**93**(6): 1210-1230. DOI: 10.1002/jcb.20284

[53] Haydon RC, Luu HH, He TC. Osteosarcoma and osteoblastic differentiation: A new perspective on oncogenesis. Clinical Orthopaedics and Related Research. 2007;**454**: 237-246. DOI: 10.1097/BLO.0b013e31802b683c

[54] Mortus JR, Zhang Y, Hughes DP. Developmental pathways hijacked by osteosarcoma. Advances in Experimental Medicine and Biology. 2014;**804**:93-118. DOI: 10.1007/978-3-319-04843-7_5

[55] Lin CH, Ji T, Chen CF, Hoang BH. Wnt signaling in osteosarcoma. Advances in Experimental Medicine and Biology. 2014;**804**:33-45. DOI: 10.1007/978-3-319-04843-7_2

[56] Li C, Shi X, Zhou G, Liu X, Wu S, Zhao J. The canonical Wnt-beta-catenin pathway in development and chemotherapy of osteosarcoma. Frontiers in Bioscience (Landmark Ed). 2013;**18**:1384-1391. http://dx.doi.org/10.2741/4187

[57] Du X, Yang J, Yang D, Tian W, Zhu Z. The genetic basis for inactivation of Wnt pathway in human osteosarcoma. BMC Cancer. 2014;**14**:450. DOI: 10.1186/1471-2407-14-450

[58] Patanè S, Avnet S, Coltella N, Costa B, Sponza S, Olivero M, et al. MET overexpression turns human primary osteoblasts into osteosarcomas. Cancer Research. 2006;**66**(9):4750-4757. DOI: 10.1158/0008-5472.CAN-05-4422

[59] Fazi B, Garbo S, Toschi N, et al. The lncRNA H19 positively affects the tumorigenic properties of glioblastoma cells and contributes to NKD1 repression through the recruitment of EZH2 on its promoter. Oncotarget. 2018;**9**(21):15512-15525. DOI: 10.18632/oncotarget.24496

[60] Li T, Zhu J, Wang X, Chen G, Sun L, Zuo S, et al. Long non-coding RNA lncTCF7 activates the Wnt/β-catenin pathway to promote metastasis and invasion in colorectal cancer. Oncology Letters. 2017;**14**(6):7384-7390. DOI: 10.3892/ol.2017.7154

[61] Wang Y, He L, Du Y, Zhu P, Huang G, Luo J, et al. The long noncoding RNA lncTCF7 promotes self-renewal of human liver cancer stem cells through activation of Wnt signaling. Cell Stem Cell. 2015;**16**(4):413-425. DOI: 10.1016/j.stem.2015.03.003

[62] Gorojankina T. Hedgehog signaling pathway: A novel model and molecular

mechanisms of signal transduction. Cellular and Molecular Life Sciences. 2016;**73**(7):1317-1332. DOI: 10.1007/s00018-015-2127-4

[63] Choudhry Z, Rikani AA, Choudhry AM, et al. Sonic hedgehog signalling pathway: A complex network. Annals of Neurosciences. 2014;**21**(1):28-31. DOI: 10.5214/ans.0972.7531.210109

[64] Armas-López L, Zúñiga J, Arrieta O, Ávila-Moreno F. The Hedgehog-GLI pathway in embryonic development and cancer: Implications for pulmonary oncology therapy. Oncotarget. 2017; **8**(36):60684-60703. DOI: 10.18632/oncotarget.19527

[65] Briscoe J, Thérond PP. The mechanisms of Hedgehog signalling and its roles in development and disease. Nature Reviews. Molecular Cell Biology. 2013;**14**(7):416-429. DOI: 10.1038/nrm3598

[66] Xavier GM, Seppala M, Barrell W, Birjandi AA, Geoghegan F, Cobourne MT. Hedgehog receptor function during craniofacial development. Developmental Biology. 2016;**415**(2): 198-215. DOI: 10.1016/j.ydbio.2016.02.009

[67] Lo WW, Pinnaduwage D, Gokgoz N, Wunder JS, Andrulis IL. Aberrant hedgehog signaling and clinical outcome in osteosarcoma. Sarcoma. 2014;**2014**: 261804. DOI: 10.1155/2014/261804

[68] Lo WW, Wunder JS, Dickson BC, Campbell V, McGovern K, Alman BA, et al. Involvement and targeted intervention of dysregulated Hedgehog signaling in osteosarcoma. Cancer. 2014; **120**(4):537-547. DOI: 10.1002/cncr.28439

[69] Chan LH, Wang W, Yeung W, Deng Y, Yuan P, Mak KK. Hedgehog signaling induces osteosarcoma development through Yap1 and H19 overexpression. Oncogene. 2014; **33**(40):4857-4866. DOI: 10.1038/onc.2013.433

[70] Verheyen EM. Opposing effects of Wnt and MAPK on BMP/Smad signal duration. Developmental Cell. 2007; **13**(6):755-756. DOI: 10.1016/j.devcel.2007.11.006

[71] Wang CL, Xiao F, Wang CD, Zhu JF, Shen C, Zuo B, et al. Gremlin2 suppression increases the BMP-2-induced osteogenesis of human bone marrow-derived mesenchymal stem cells via the BMP-2/Smad/Runx2 signaling pathway. Journal of Cellular Biochemistry. 2017;**118**(2):286-297. DOI: 10.1002/jcb.25635

[72] Rahman MS, Akhtar N, Jamil HM, Banik RS, Asaduzzaman SM. TGF-β/BMP signaling and other molecular events: Regulation of osteoblastogenesis and bone formation. Bone Research. 2015;**3**:15005. DOI: 10.1038/boneres.2015.5

[73] Chen G, Deng C, Li YP. TGF-β and BMP signaling in osteoblast differentiation and bone formation. International Journal of Biological Sciences. 2012;**8**(2):272-288. DOI: 10.7150/ijbs.2929

[74] Zuo C, Wang Z, Lu H, Dai Z, Liu X, Cui L. Expression profiling of lncRNAs in C3H10T1/2 mesenchymal stem cells undergoing early osteoblast differentiation. Molecular Medicine Reports. 2013 Aug;**8**(2):463-467. DOI: 10.3892/mmr.2013.1540

[75] Zhu L, Xu PC. Downregulated LncRNA-ANCR promotes osteoblast differentiation by targeting EZH2 and regulating Runx2 expression. Biochemical and Biophysical Research Communications. 2013; **432**(4):612-617. DOI: 10.1016/j.bbrc.2013.02.036

[76] Nguyen A, Scott MA, Dry SM, James AW. Roles of bone morphogenetic protein signaling in

osteosarcoma. International Orthopaedics. 2014;**38**(11):2313-2322. DOI: 10.1007/s00264-014-2512-x

[77] Wang S, Ren T, Jiao G, et al. BMPR2 promotes invasion and metastasis via the RhoA-ROCK-LIMK2 pathway in human osteosarcoma cells. Oncotarget. 2017;**8**(35):58625-58641. DOI: 10.18632/oncotarget.17382

[78] Guan G, Zhang Y, Lu Y, Liu L, Shi D, Wen Y, et al. The HIF-1α/CXCR4 pathway supports hypoxia-induced metastasis of human osteosarcoma cells. Cancer Letters. 2015;**357**(1):254-264. DOI: 10.1016/j.canlet.2014.11.034

[79] Zhao H, Wu Y, Chen Y, Liu H. Clinical significance of hypoxia-inducible factor 1 and VEGF-A in osteosarcoma. International Journal of Clinical Oncology. 2015;**20**(6):1233-1243. DOI: 10.1007/s10147-015-0848-x

[80] Wang Y, Yao J, Meng H, et al. A novel long non-coding RNA, hypoxia-inducible factor-2α promoter upstream transcript, functions as an inhibitor of osteosarcoma stem cells in vitro. Molecular Medicine Reports. 2014;**11**(4):2534-2540. DOI: 10.3892/mmr.2014.3024

[81] Xu Y, Wang S, Tang C, Chen W. Upregulation of long non-coding RNA HIF 1α-anti-sense 1 induced by transforming growth factor-β-mediated targeting of sirtuin 1 promotes osteoblastic differentiation of human bone marrow stromal cells. Molecular Medicine Reports. 2015;**12**(5):7233-7238. DOI: 10.3892/mmr.2015.4415

[82] Tao J, Jiang MM, Jiang L, et al. Notch activation as a driver of osteogenic sarcoma. Cancer Cell. 2014;**26**(3):390-401. DOI: 10.1016/j.ccr.2014.07.023

[83] Li YS, Deng ZH, Zeng C, Lei GH. JNK pathway in osteosarcoma: Pathogenesis and therapeutics. Journal of Receptor and Signal Transduction Research. 2016;**36**(5):465-470. DOI: 10.3109/10799893.2015.1122045

[84] Zhang J, Yu XH, Yan YG, Wang C, Wang WJ. PI3K/Akt signaling in osteosarcoma. Clinica Chimica Acta. 2015;**444**:182-192. DOI: 10.1016/j.cca.2014.12.041

[85] Adamopoulos C, Gargalionis AN, Basdra EK, Papavassiliou AG. Deciphering signaling networks in osteosarcoma pathobiology. Experimental Biology and Medicine (Maywood, N.J.). 2016;**241**(12):1296-1305. DOI: 10.1177/1535370216648806

[86] Li JP, Liu LH, Li J, Chen Y, Jiang XW, Ouyang YR, et al. Microarray expression profile of long noncoding RNAs in human osteosarcoma. Biochemical and Biophysical Research Communications. 2013;**433**(2):200-206. DOI: 10.1016/j.bbrc.2013.02.083

[87] Dong Y, Liang G, Yuan B, Yang C, Gao R, Zhou X. MALAT1 promotes the proliferation and metastasis of osteosarcoma cells by activating the PI3K/Akt pathway. Tumour Biology. 2015;**36**(3):1477-1486. DOI: 10.1007/s13277-014-2631-4

[88] Cai X, Liu Y, Yang W, Xia Y, Yang C, Yang S, et al. Long noncoding RNA MALAT1 as a potential therapeutic target in osteosarcoma. Journal of Orthopaedic Research. 2016;**34**(6):932-941. DOI: 10.1002/jor.23105

[89] Qian M, Yang X, Li Z, Jiang C, Song D, Yan W, et al. P50-associated COX-2 extragenic RNA (PACER) overexpression promotes proliferation and metastasis of osteosarcoma cells by activating COX-2 gene. Tumour Biology. 2016;**37**(3):3879-3886. DOI: 10.1007/s13277-015-3838-8

[90] Feng ZM, Guo SM. Tim-3 facilitates osteosarcoma proliferation and metastasis through the NF-κB pathway and epithelial-mesenchymal transition.

Genetics and Molecular Research. 2016;**15**(3):7844. DOI: 10.4238/gmr.15037844

[91] Gong T, Su X, Xia Q, Wang J, Kan S. Expression of NF-κB and PTEN in osteosarcoma and its clinical significance. Oncology Letters. 2017; **14**(6):6744-6748. DOI: 10.3892/ol.2017.6972

[92] Arshad A, Lifang H, Airong Q, Chu C, Tuanmin Y. Long noncoding RNAs and human osteosarcoma. Journal of Stem Cell Research and Therapy. 2018; **8**(3):418. DOI: 10.4172/2157-7633.1000418

[93] Gabory A, Jammes H, Dandolo L. The H19 locus: Role of an imprinted non-coding RNA in growth and development. BioEssays. 2010;**32**: 473-480. DOI: 10.1002/bies.200900170

[94] Berteaux N, Aptel N, Cathala G, et al. A novel H19 antisense RNA overexpressed in breast cancer contributes to paternal IGF2 expression. Molecular and Cellular Biology. 2008; **28**(22):6731-6745. DOI: 10.1128/MCB.02103-07

[95] Tran VG, Court F, Duputié A, et al. H19 antisense RNA can up-regulate IGF2 transcription by activation of a novel promoter in mouse myoblasts. PLoS One. 2012;**7**(5):e37923. DOI: 10.1371/journal.pone.0037923

[96] Dunn KL, Davie JR. The many roles of the transcriptional regulator CTCF. Biochemistry and Cell Biology. 2003;**81**(3):161-167. DOI: 10.1139/o03-052

[97] Ulaner GA, Vu TH, Li T, Hu JF, Yao XM, Yang Y, et al. Loss of imprinting of IGF2 and H19 in osteosarcoma is accompanied by reciprocal methylation changes of a CTCF-binding site. Human Molecular Genetics. 2003;**12**(5):535-549. DOI: 10.1093/hmg/ddg034

[98] Xia WK, Lin QF, Shen D, Liu ZL, Su J, Mao WD. Clinical implication of long noncoding RNA 91H expression profile in osteosarcoma patients. OncoTargets and Therapy. 2016;**9**:4645-4652. DOI: 10.2147/OTT.S103376

[99] Zhu L, Xu PC. Downregulated LncRNA-ANCR promotes osteoblast differentiation by targeting EZH2 and regulating Runx2 expression. Biochemical Biophysical Research Communications. 2013;**432**(4):612-617. DOI: 10.1016/j.bbrc.2013.02.036

[100] Zhang F, Peng H. LncRNA-ANCR regulates the cell growth of osteosarcoma by interacting with EZH2 and affecting the expression of p21 and p27. Journal of Orthopaedic Surgery and Research. 2017;**12**(1):103. DOI: 10.1186/s13018-017-0599-7

[101] Min L, Hong S, Duan H, Zhou Y, Zhang W, Luo Y, et al. Antidifferentiation noncoding RNA regulates the proliferation of osteosarcoma cells. Cancer Biotherapy & Radiopharmaceuticals. 2016;**31**(2):52-57. DOI: 10.1089/cbr.2015.1888

[102] Godinho M, Meijer D, Setyono-Han B, Dorssers LC, van Agthoven T. Characterization of BCAR4, a novel oncogene causing endocrine resistance in human breast cancer cells. Journal of Cellular Physiology. 2011;**226**(7): 1741-1749. DOI: 10.1002/jcp.22503

[103] Godinho MF, Sieuwerts AM, Look MP, et al. Relevance of BCAR4 in tamoxifen resistance and tumour aggressiveness of human breast cancer. British Journal of Cancer. 2010;**103**(8): 1284-1291. DOI: 10.1038/sj.bjc.6605884

[104] Chen F, Mo J, Zhang L. Long noncoding RNA BCAR4 promotes osteosarcoma progression through activating GLI2-dependent gene transcription. Tumour Biology. 2016; **37**(10):13403-13412. DOI: 10.1007/s13277-016-5256-y

[105] Ju L, Zhou YM, Yang GS. Up-regulation of long non-coding RNA BCAR4 predicts a poor prognosis in patients with osteosarcoma, and promotes cell invasion and metastasis. European Review for Medical and Pharmacological Sciences. 2016;**20**(21): 4445-4451

[106] Li Z, Dou P, Liu T, He S. Application of long noncoding RNAs in osteosarcoma: biomarkers and therapeutic targets. Cellular Physiology and Biochemistry. 2017;**42**(4): 1407-1419. DOI: 10.1159/000479205

[107] Sun J, Wang X, Fu C, Zou J, Hua H, Bi Z. Long noncoding RNA FGFR3-AS1 promotes osteosarcoma growth through regulating its natural antisense transcript FGFR3. Molecular Biology Reports. 2016;**43**:427-436. DOI: 10.1007/s11033-016-3975-1

[108] Li W, He X, Xue R, Zhang Y, Zhang X, Lu J, et al. Combined over-expression of the hypoxia-inducible factor 2α gene and its long non-coding RNA predicts unfavorable prognosis of patients with osteosarcoma. Pathology, Research and Practice. 2016;**212**: 861-866. DOI: 10.1016/j.prp.2016. 06.013

[109] Preker P, Almvig K, Christensen MS, Valen E, Mapendano CK, Sandelin A, et al. PROMoter uPstream transcripts share characteristics with mRNAs and are produced upstream of all three major types of mammalian promoters. Nucleic Acids Research. 2011;**39**:7179-7193. DOI: 10.1093/nar/gkr370

[110] Taft RJ, Kaplan CD, Simons C, Mattick JS. Evolution, biogenesis and function of promoter-associated RNAs. Cell Cycle. 2009;**8**:2332-2338. DOI: 10.4161/cc.8.15.9154

[111] Albrecht AS, Ørom UA. Bidirectional expression of long ncRNA/protein-coding gene pairs in cancer. Briefings in Functional Genomics. 2016;**15**(3):167-173. DOI: 10.1093/bfgp/elv048

[112] Yao J, Li J, Geng P, Li Y, Chen H, Zhu Y. Knockdown of a HIF-2alpha promoter upstream long noncoding RNA impairs colorectal cancer stem cell properties in vitro through HIF-2alpha downregulation. OncoTargets and Therapy. 2015;**8**:3467-3474. DOI: 10.2147/OTT.S81393

[113] Wang B, Su Y, Yang Q, Lv D, Zhang W, Tang K, et al. Overexpression of long non-coding RNA HOTAIR promotes tumor growth and metastasis in human osteosarcoma. Molecules and Cells. 2015;**38**(5):432-440. DOI: 10.14348/molcells.2015.2327

[114] Qiu JJ, Lin YY, Ye LC, Ding JX, Feng WW, Jin HY, et al. Overexpression of long non-coding RNA HOTAIR predicts poor patient prognosis and promotes tumor metastasis in epithelial ovarian cancer. Gynecologic Oncology. 2014;**134**(1):121-128. DOI: 10.1016/j.ygyno.2014.03.556

[115] Liu XH, Liu ZL, Sun M, Liu J, Wang ZX, De W. The long non-coding RNA HOTAIR indicates a poor prognosis and promotes metastasis in non-small cell lung cancer. BMC Cancer. 2013;**13**:464. DOI: 10.1186/1471-2407-13-464

[116] Xue X, Yang YA, Zhang A, et al. LncRNA HOTAIR enhances ER signaling and confers tamoxifen resistance in breast cancer. Oncogene. 2015;**35**(21):2746-2755. DOI: 10.1038/onc.2015.340

[117] Wu L, Zhang L, Zheng S. Role of the long non-coding RNA HOTAIR in hepatocellular carcinoma. Oncology Letters. 2017;**14**(2):1233-1239. DOI: 10.3892/ol.2017.6312

[118] Zhang J, Zhang P, Wang L, Piao HL, Ma L. Long non-coding RNA

HOTAIR in carcinogenesis and metastasis. Acta Biochimica et Biophysica Sinica Shanghai. 2013;**46**(1): 1-5. DOI: 10.1093/abbs/gmt117

[119] Tsai MC, Manor O, Wan Y, et al. Long noncoding RNA as modular scaffold of histone modification complexes. Science. 2010;**329**(5992): 689-693. DOI: 10.1126/science.1192002

[120] Zhou Q, Chen F, Fei Z, et al. Genetic variants of lncRNA HOTAIR contribute to the risk of osteosarcoma. Oncotarget. 2016;**7**(15):19928-19934. DOI: 10.18632/oncotarget.7957

[121] Li F, Cao L, Hang D, Wang F, Wang Q. Long non-coding RNA HOTTIP is up-regulated and associated with poor prognosis in patients with osteosarcoma. International Journal of Clinical and Experimental Pathology. 2015;**8**(9):11414-11420

[122] Cheng Y, Jutooru I, Chadalapaka G, Corton JC, Safe S. The long non-coding RNA HOTTIP enhances pancreatic cancer cell proliferation, survival and migration. Oncotarget. 2015;**6**(13): 10840-10852. DOI: 10.18632/oncotarget.3450

[123] Ye H, Liu K, Qian K. Overexpression of long noncoding RNA HOTTIP promotes tumor invasion and predicts poor prognosis in gastric cancer. OncoTargets and Therapy. 2016; **9**:2081-2088. DOI: 10.2147/OTT.S95414

[124] Chen X, Han H, Li Y, Zhang Q, Mo K, Chen S. Upregulation of long noncoding RNA HOTTIP promotes metastasis of esophageal squamous cell carcinoma via induction of EMT. Oncotarget. 2016;**7**(51):84480-84485. DOI: 10.18632/oncotarget.12995

[125] Zhang GJ, Song W, Song Y. Overexpression of HOTTIP promotes proliferation and drug resistance of lung adenocarcinoma by regulating AKT signaling pathway. European Review for Medical and Pharmacological Sciences. 2017;**21**(24):5683-5690. DOI: 10.26355/eurrev_201712_14013

[126] Wang KC, Yang YW, Liu B, et al. A long noncoding RNA maintains active chromatin to coordinate homeotic gene expression. Nature. 2011;**472**(7341): 120-124. DOI: 10.1038/nature09819

[127] Lian Y, Cai Z, Gong H, Xue S, Wu D, Wang K. HOTTIP: A critical oncogenic long non-coding RNA in human cancers. Molecular BioSystems. 2016;**12**(11):3247-3253. DOI: 10.1039/c6mb00475j

[128] Li Z, Yu X, Shen J. Long non-coding RNAs: Emerging players in osteosarcoma. Tumour Biology. 2016 Mar;**37**(3):2811-2816. DOI: 10.1007/s13277-015-4749-4

[129] Yu X, Zheng H, Chan MT, Wu WK. HULC: An oncogenic long non-coding RNA in human cancer. Journal of Cellular and Molecular Medicine. 2016; **21**(2):410-417. DOI: 10.1111/jcmm.12956

[130] Hämmerle M, Gutschner T, Uckelmann H, Ozgur S, Fiskin E, Gross M, et al. Posttranscriptional destabilization of the liver-specific long noncoding RNA HULC by the IGF2 mRNA-binding protein 1 (IGF2BP1). Hepatology. 2013;**58**(5):1703-1712. DOI: 10.1002/hep.26537

[131] Cui M, Xiao Z, Wang Y, Zheng M, Song T, Cai X, et al. Long noncoding RNA HULC modulates abnormal lipid metabolism in hepatoma cells through an miR-9-mediated RXRA signaling pathway. Cancer Research. 2015;**75**(5): 846-857. DOI: 10.1158/0008-5472.CAN-14-1192

[132] Li SP, Xu HX, Yu Y, et al. LncRNA HULC enhances epithelial-mesenchymal transition to promote tumorigenesis and metastasis of hepatocellular carcinoma via the

miR-200a-3p/ZEB1 signaling pathway. Oncotarget. 2016;7(27):42431-42446. DOI: 10.18632/oncotarget.9883

[133] Yang XJ, Huang CQ, Peng CW, Hou JX, Liu JY. Long noncoding RNA HULC promotes colorectal carcinoma progression through epigenetically repressing NKD2 expression. Gene. 2016;**592**(1):172-178. DOI: 10.1016/j.gene.2016.08.002

[134] Lu Z, Xiao Z, Liu F, et al. Long non-coding RNA HULC promotes tumor angiogenesis in liver cancer by up-regulating sphingosine kinase 1 (SPHK1). Oncotarget. 2015;7(1): 241-254. DOI: 10.18632/oncotarget.6280

[135] Sun XH, Yang LB, Geng XL, Wang R, Zhang ZC. Increased expression of lncRNA HULC indicates a poor prognosis and promotes cell metastasis in osteosarcoma. International Journal of Clinical and Experimental Pathology. 2015;**8**(3):2994-3000

[136] Uzan VR, Av L, Boldrini É, et al. High expression of HULC is associated with poor prognosis in osteosarcoma patients. PLoS One. 2016;**11**(6): e0156774. DOI: 10.1371/journal.pone.0156774

[137] Ji P, Diederichs S, Wang W, Böing S, Metzger R, Schneider PM, et al. MALAT-1, a novel noncoding RNA, and thymosin beta4 predict metastasis and survival in early-stage non-small cell lung cancer. Oncogene. 2003;**22**(39): 8031-8041. DOI: 10.1038/sj.onc.1206928

[138] Gutschner T, Hämmerle M, Eissmann M, et al. The noncoding RNA MALAT1 is a critical regulator of the metastasis phenotype of lung cancer cells. Cancer Research. 2012;**73**(3): 1180-1189. DOI: 10.1158/0008-5472.CAN-12-2850

[139] Chou J, Wang B, Zheng T, Li X, Zheng L, Hu J, et al. MALAT1 induced migration and invasion of human breast cancer cells by competitively binding miR-1 with cdc42. Biochemical and Biophysical Research Communications. 2016;**472**(1):262-269. DOI: 10.1016/j.bbrc.2016.02.102

[140] Li J, Wang J, Chen Y, et al. LncRNA MALAT1 exerts oncogenic functions in lung adenocarcinoma by targeting miR-204. American Journal of Cancer Research. 2016;**6**(5):1099-1107

[141] Luan W, Li L, Shi Y, et al. Long non-coding RNA MALAT1 acts as a competing endogenous RNA to promote malignant melanoma growth and metastasis by sponging miR-22. Oncotarget. 2016;7(39):63901-63912. DOI: 10.18632/oncotarget.11564

[142] Huo Y, Li Q, Wang X, et al. MALAT1 predicts poor survival in osteosarcoma patients and promotes cell metastasis through associating with EZH2. Oncotarget. 2017;**8**(29): 46993-47006. DOI: 10.18632/oncotarget.16551

[143] Chen D, Wang H, Zhang M, Jiang S, Zhou C, Fang B, et al. Abnormally expressed long non-coding RNAs in prognosis of Osteosarcoma: A systematic review and meta-analysis. Journal of Bone Oncology. 2018;**13**: 76-90. DOI: 10.1016/j.jbo.2018.09.005

[144] Luo W, He H, Xiao W, et al. MALAT1 promotes osteosarcoma development by targeting TGFA via MIR376A. Oncotarget. 2016;7(34): 54733-54743. DOI: 10.18632/oncotarget.10752

[145] Taniguchi M, Fujiwara K, Nakai Y, et al. Inhibition of malignant phenotypes of human osteosarcoma cells by a gene silencer, a pyrrole-imidazole polyamide, which targets an E-box motif. FEBS Open Bio. 2014;**4**:328-334. DOI: 10.1016/j.fob.2014. 03.004

[146] Li Z, Shen J, Chan MT, Wu WK. TUG1: A pivotal oncogenic long

non-coding RNA of human cancers. Cell Proliferation. 2016;**49**(4):471-475. DOI: 10.1111/cpr.12269

[147] Khalil AM, Guttman M, Huarte M, et al. Many human large intergenic noncoding RNAs associate with chromatin-modifying complexes and affect gene expression. Proceedings of the National Academy of Sciences of the United States of America. 2009;**106**(28): 11667-11672. DOI: 10.1073/pnas.0904715106

[148] Xie CH, Cao YM, Huang Y, Shi QW, Guo JH, Fan ZW, et al. Long non-coding RNA TUG1 contributes to tumorigenesis of human osteosarcoma by sponging miR-9-5p and regulating POU2F1 expression. Tumour Biology. 2016 Nov;**37**(11):15031-15041. DOI: 10.1007/s13277-016-5391-5

[149] Cao J, Han X, Qi X, Jin X, Li X. TUG1 promotes osteosarcoma tumorigenesis by upregulating EZH2 expression via miR-144-3p. International Journal of Oncology. 2017; **51**(4):1115-1123. DOI: 10.3892/ijo.2017.4110

[150] Li H, Tian G, Tian F, Shao L. Long non-coding RNA TUG1 promotes osteosarcoma cell proliferation and invasion through inhibition of microRNA-212-3p expression. Experimental and Therapeutic Medicine. 2018;**16**(2):779-787. DOI: 10.3892/etm.2018.6216

[151] Zhang Q, Geng PL, Yin P, Wang XL, Jia JP, Yao J. Down-regulation of long non-coding RNA TUG1 inhibits osteosarcoma cell proliferation and promotes apoptosis. Asian Pacific Journal of Cancer Prevention. 2013; **14**(4):2311-2315. DOI: 10.7314/APJCP.2013.14.4.2311

[152] Ma B, Li M, Zhang L, Huang M, Lei JB, Fu GH, et al. Upregulation of long non-coding RNA TUG1 correlates with poor prognosis and disease status in osteosarcoma. Tumour Biology. 2016; (4):4445-4455. DOI: 10.1007/s13277-015-4301-6

[153] Jin B, Gong Y, Li H, Jiao L, Xin D, Gong Y, et al. C/EBPβ promotes the viability of human bladder cancer cell by contributing to the transcription of bladder cancer specific lncRNA UCA1. Biochemical and Biophysical Research Communications. 2018; pii: S0006-291X(18)32330-1. DOI: 10.1016/j.bbrc.2018.10.152

[154] Xue M, Chen W, Li X. Urothelial cancer associated 1: A long noncoding RNA with a crucial role in cancer. Journal of Cancer Research and Clinical Oncology. 2016;**142**:1407-1419. DOI: 10.1007/s00432-015-2042-y

[155] He A, Hu R, Chen Z, et al. Role of long noncoding RNA UCA1 as a common molecular marker for lymph node metastasis and prognosis in various cancers: A meta-analysis. Oncotarget. 2016;**8**(1):1937-1943. DOI: 10.18632/oncotarget.12463

[156] Liu FT, Zhu PQ, Luo HL, Zhang Y, Qiu C. Prognostic value of long non-coding RNA UCA1 in human solid tumors. Oncotarget. 2016;**7**(36):57991-58000. DOI: 10.18632/oncotarget. 11155

[157] Wang X, Gong Y, Jin B, et al. Long non-coding RNA urothelial carcinoma associated 1 induces cell replication by inhibiting BRG1 in 5637 cells. Oncology Reports. 2014;**32**(3):1281-1290. DOI: 10.3892/or.2014.3309

[158] Wang F, Ying HQ, He BS, et al. Upregulated lncRNA-UCA1 contributes to progression of hepatocellular carcinoma through inhibition of miR-216b and activation of FGFR1/ERK signaling pathway. Oncotarget. 2015; **6**(10):7899-7917. DOI: 10.18632/oncotarget.3219

[159] Sun X, Haider Ali MSS, Moran M. The role of interactions of long

non-coding RNAs and heterogeneous nuclear ribonucleoproteins in regulating cellular functions. The Biochemical Journal. 2017;**474**(17):2925-2935. DOI: 10.1042/BCJ20170280

[160] Li T, Xiao Y, Huang T. HIF-1α-induced upregulation of lncRNA UCA1 promotes cell growth in osteosarcoma by inactivating the PTEN/AKT signaling pathway. Oncology Reports. 2018;**39**(3): 1072-1080. DOI: 10.3892/or.2018.6182

[161] Li C, Liang G, Yang S, et al. Dysregulated lncRNA-UCA1 contributes to the progression of gastric cancer through regulation of the PI3K-Akt-mTOR signaling pathway. Oncotarget. 2017;**8**(55):93476-93491. DOI: 10.18632/oncotarget.19281

[162] Shao Y, Li H, Du R, Meng J, Yang G. Involvement of non-coding RNAs in chemotherapy resistance of ovarian cancer. Journal of Cancer. 2018;**9**(11): 1966-1972. Published 2018 Ap. 30. DOI: 10.7150/jca.24550

[163] Wang H, Guan Z, He K, Qian J, Cao J, Teng L. LncRNA UCA1 in anti-cancer drug resistance. Oncotarget. 2017;**8**(38):64638-64650. DOI: 10.18632/oncotarget.18344

[164] Liu H, Wang G, Yang L, Qu J, Yang Z, Zhou X. Knockdown of long non-coding RNA UCA1 increases the tamoxifen sensitivity of breast cancer cells through inhibition of Wnt/β-catenin pathway. PLoS One. 2016; **11**(12):e0168406. DOI: 10.1371/journal.pone.0168406

[165] Li W, Xie P, Ruan WH. Overexpression of lncRNA UCA1 promotes osteosarcoma progression and correlates with poor prognosis. Journal of Bone Oncology. 2016;**5**(2):80-85. DOI: 10.1016/j.jbo.2016.05.003

[166] Yin Z, Ding H, He E, Chen J, Li M. Overexpression of long non-coding RNA MFI2 promotes cell proliferation and suppresses apoptosis in human osteosarcoma. Oncology Reports. 2016; **36**(4):2033-2040. DOI: 10.3892/or.2016.5013

[167] Ruan W, Wang P, Feng S, Xue Y, Li Y. Long non-coding RNA small nucleolar RNA host gene 12 (SNHG12) promotes cell proliferation and migration by upregulating angiomotin gene expression in human osteosarcoma cells. Tumour Biology. 2016;**37**(3): 4065-4073. DOI: 10.1007/s13277-015-4256-7

[168] Zhou S, Yu L, Xiong M, Dai G. LncRNA SNHG12 promotes tumorigenesis and metastasis in osteosarcoma by upregulating Notch2 by sponging miR-195-5p. Biochemical and Biophysical Research Communications. 2018;**495**(2):1822-1832. DOI: 10.1016/j.bbrc.2017.12.047

[169] Liu C, Lin J. Long noncoding RNA ZEB1-AS1 acts as an oncogene in osteosarcoma by epigenetically activating ZEB1. American Journal of Translational Research. 2016;**8**(10): 4095-4105

[170] Liu C, Pan C, Cai Y, Wang H. Interplay between long noncoding RNA ZEB1-AS1 and miR-200s regulates osteosarcoma cell proliferation and migration. Journal of Cellular Biochemistry. 2017;**118**(8):2250-2260. DOI: 10.1002/jcb.25879

[171] Pasic I, Shlien A, Durbin AD, Stavropoulos DJ, Baskin B, Ray PN, et al. Recurrent focal copy-number changes and loss of heterozygosity implicate two noncoding RNAs and one tumor suppressor gene at chromosome 3q13.31 in osteosarcoma. Cancer Research. 2010;**70**:160-171. DOI: 10.1158/0008-5472.CAN-09-1902

[172] Xie J, Lin D, Lee DH, Akunowicz J, Hansen M, Miller C, et al. Copy number analysis identifies tumor suppressive lncRNAs in human osteosarcoma.

International Journal of Oncology. 2017; **50**(3):863-872. DOI: 10.3892/ijo.2017.3864

[173] Liu Q, Huang J, Zhou N, et al. LncRNA loc285194 is a p53-regulated tumor suppressor. Nucleic Acids Research. 2013;**41**(9):4976-4987. DOI: 10.1093/nar/gkt182

[174] Zhang A, Xu M, Mo YY. Role of the lncRNA-p53 regulatory network in cancer. Journal of Molecular Cell Biology. 2014;**6**(3):181-191. DOI: 10.1093/jmcb/mju013

[175] Salmena L, Poliseno L, Tay Y, Kats L, Pandolfi PP. A ceRNA hypothesis: The Rosetta Stone of a hidden RNA language? Cell. 2011;**146**(3):353-358. DOI: 10.1016/j.cell.2011.07.014

[176] da Rocha ST, Edwards CA, Ito M, Ogata T, Ferguson-Smith AC. Genomic imprinting at the mammalian Dlk1-Dio3 domain.Trends in Genetics 2008;**24**(6): 306-316. DOI: 10.1016/j.tig.2008.03.011

[177] He Y, Luo Y, Liang B, Ye L, Lu G, He W. Potential applications of MEG3 in cancer diagnosis and prognosis. Oncotarget. 2017;**8**(42):73282-73295. DOI: 10.18632/oncotarget.19931

[178] Zhou Y, Zhang X, Klibanski A. MEG3 noncoding RNA: A tumor suppressor. Journal of Molecular Endocrinology. 2012;**48**(3):R45-R53. DOI: 10.1530/JME-12-0008

[179] Zhu M, Wang X, Gu Y, Wang F, Li L, Qiu X. MEG3 overexpression inhibits the tumorigenesis of breast cancer by downregulating miR-21 through the PI3K/Akt pathway. Archives of Biochemistry and Biophysics. 2018;**661**: 22-30. DOI: 10.1016/j.abb.2018.10.021

[180] Zhang CY, Yu MS, Li X, Zhang Z, Han CR, Yan B. Overexpression of long non-coding RNA MEG3 suppresses breast cancer cell proliferation, invasion, and angiogenesis through AKT pathway. Tumour Biology. 2017;**39**(6): 1-12. DOI: 10.1177/1010428317701311

[181] He JH, Han ZP, Liu JM, Zhou JB, Zou MX, Lv YB, et al. Overexpression of long non-coding RNA MEG3 inhibits proliferation of hepatocellular carcinoma Huh7 Cells via negative modulation of miRNA-664. Journal of Cellular Biochemistry. 2017;**118**(11): 3713-3721. DOI: 10.1002/jcb.26018

[182] Sun L, Li Y, Yang B. Downregulated long non-coding RNA MEG3 in breast cancer regulates proliferation, migration and invasion by depending on p53's transcriptional activity. Biochemical and Biophysical Research Communications. 2016; **478**(1):323-329. DOI: 10.1016/j.bbrc.2016.05.031

[183] Zhang J, Yao T, Wang Y, Yu J, Liu Y, Lin Z. Long noncoding RNA MEG3 is downregulated in cervical cancer and affects cell proliferation and apoptosis by regulating miR-21. Cancer Biology & Therapy. 2015;**17**(1): 104-113. DOI: 10.1080/15384047.2015.1108496

[184] Lu KH, Li W, Liu XH, et al. Long non-coding RNA MEG3 inhibits NSCLC cells proliferation and induces apoptosis by affecting p53 expression. BMC Cancer. 2013;**13**:461. DOI: 10.1186/1471-2407-13-461

[185] Liu Z, Wu C, Xie N, Wang P. Long non-coding RNA MEG3 inhibits the proliferation and metastasis of oral squamous cell carcinoma by regulating the WNT/β-catenin signaling pathway. Oncology Letters. 2017;**14**(4): 4053-4058. DOI: 10.3892/ol.2017.6682

[186] Zarkou V, Galaras A, Giakountis A, Hatzis P. Crosstalk mechanisms between the WNT signaling pathway and long non-coding RNAs. Non-coding RNA Research. 2018;**3**(2):42-53. DOI: 10.1016/j.ncrna.2018.04.001

[187] Shi Y, Lv C, Shi L, Tu G. MEG3 inhibits proliferation and invasion and promotes apoptosis of human osteosarcoma cells. Oncology Letters. 2018;**15**(2):1917-1923. DOI: 10.3892/ol.2017.7463

[188] Tian ZZ, Guo XJ, Zhao YM, Fang Y. Decreased expression of long non-coding RNA MEG3 acts as a potential predictor biomarker in progression and poor prognosis of osteosarcoma. International Journal of Clinical and Experimental Pathology. 2015;**8**(11): 15138-15142

[189] Li N, Shi K, Li W. TUSC7: A novel tumor suppressor long non-coding RNA in human cancers. Journal of Cellular Physiology. 2018;**233**(9):6401-6407. DOI: 10.1002/jcp.26544

[190] Cong M, Li J, Jing R, Li Z. Long non-coding RNA tumor suppressor candidate 7 functions as a tumor suppressor and inhibits proliferation in osteosarcoma. Tumour Biology. 2016; **37**(7):9441-9450. DOI: 10.1007/s13277-015-4414-y

[191] Celià-Terrassa T, Kang Y. Distinctive properties of metastasis-initiating cells. Genes & Development. 2016;**30**(8):892-908. DOI: 10.1101/gad.277681.116

[192] Hurst DR, Welch DR. Metastasis suppressor genes at the interface between the environment and tumor cell growth. International Review of Cell and Molecular Biology. 2011;**286**: 107-180. DOI: 10.1016/B978-0-12-385859-7.00003-3

[193] Malagobadan S, Nagoor NH. Evaluation of MicroRNAs regulating anoikis pathways and its therapeutic potential. BioMed Research International. 2015;**2015**:716816. DOI: 10.1155/2015/716816

[194] Cao Z, Livas T, Kyprianou N. Anoikis and EMT: Lethal "Liaisons" during cancer progression. Critical Reviews in Oncogenesis. 2016;**21**(3–4): 155-168. DOI: 10.1615/CritRevOncog.2016016955

[195] Li J, Yang Z, Li Y, et al. Cell apoptosis, autophagy and necroptosis in osteosarcoma treatment. Oncotarget. 2016;**7**(28):44763-44778. DOI: 10.18632/oncotarget.8206

[196] Maugg D, Rothenaigner I, Schorpp K, et al. New small molecules targeting apoptosis and cell viability in osteosarcoma. PLoS One. 2015;**10**(6): e0129058. DOI: 10.1371/journal.pone.0129058

[197] He P, Zhang Z, Huang G, et al. miR-141 modulates osteoblastic cell proliferation by regulating the target gene of lncRNA H19 and lncRNA H19-derived miR-675. American Journal of Translational Research. 2016;**8**(4): 1780-1788

[198] Peng ZQ, Lu RB, Xiao DM, Xiao ZM. Increased expression of the lncRNA BANCR and its prognostic significance in human osteosarcoma. Genetics and Molecular Research. 2016;**15**(1):7480. DOI: 10.4238/gmr.15017480

[199] Sun Y, Qin B. Long noncoding RNA MALAT1 regulates HDAC4-mediated proliferation and apoptosis via decoying of miR-140-5p in osteosarcoma cells. Cancer Medicine. 2018;**7**(9):4584-4597. DOI: 10.1002/cam4.1677

[200] Liu Q, Zhang H, Jiang X, Qian C, Liu Z, Luo D. Factors involved in cancer metastasis: A better understanding to "seed and soil" hypothesis. Molecular Cancer. 2017;**16**(1):176. DOI: 176. DOI: 10.1186/s12943-017-0742-4

[201] Lambert AW, Pattabiraman DR, Weinberg RA. Emerging biological principles of metastasis. Cell. 2017; **168**(4):670-691. DOI: 10.1016/j.cell.2016.11.037

[202] Jiang C, Li X, Zhao H, Liu H. Long non-coding RNAs: Potential new biomarkers for predicting tumor invasion and metastasis. Molecular Cancer. 2016;**15**(1):62. DOI: 10.1186/s12943-016-0545-z

[203] Xie L, Yao Z, Zhang Y, et al. Deep RNA sequencing reveals the dynamic regulation of miRNA, lncRNAs, and mRNAs in osteosarcoma tumorigenesis and pulmonary metastasis. Cell Death & Disease. 2018;**9**(7):772. DOI: 10.1038/s41419-018-0813-5

[204] Gong J, Zhang H, He L, Wang L, Wang J. Increased expression of long non-coding RNA BCAR4 is predictive of poor prognosis in patients with non-small cell lung cancer. The Tohoku Journal of Experimental Medicine. 2017;**241**(1):29-34. DOI: 10.1620/tjem.241.29

[205] Xing Z, Lin C, Yang L. Unraveling the therapeutic potential of the LncRNA-dependent noncanonical Hedgehog pathway in cancer. Molecular & Cellular Oncology. 2015;**2**(4):e998900. DOI: 10.1080/23723556.2014.998900

[206] Wang Y, Zeng X, Wang N, et al. Long noncoding RNA DANCR, working as a competitive endogenous RNA, promotes ROCK1-mediated proliferation and metastasis via decoying of miR-335-5p and miR-1972 in osteosarcoma. Molecular Cancer. 2018;**17**(1):89. DOI: 10.1186/s12943-018-0837-6

[207] Wang B, Su Y, Yang Q, Lv D, Zhang W, Tang K, Wang H, Zhang R, Liu R. Overexpression of long non-Coding RNA HOTAIR promotes tumor growth and metastasis in human osteosarcoma. Molecules and Cells 2015;**38**(5):432-440. DOI: 10.14348/molcells.2015.2327

[208] Xiao H, Zhang F, Zou Y, Li J, Liu Y, Huang W. The function and mechanism of long non-coding RNA-ATB in cancers. Frontiers in Physiology. 2018;**9**:321. DOI: 10.3389/fphys.2018.00321

[209] Burk U, Schubert J, Wellner U, et al. A reciprocal repression between ZEB1 and members of the miR-200 family promotes EMT and invasion in cancer cells. EMBO Reports. 2008;**9**(6):582-589. DOI: 10.1038/embor.2008.74

[210] Jang SY, Kim G, Park SY, et al. Clinical significance of lncRNA-ATB expression in human hepatocellular carcinoma. Oncotarget. 2017;**8**(45):78588-78597. DOI: 10.18632/oncotarget.21094

[211] Yuan JH, Yang F, Wang F, Ma JZ, Guo YJ, Tao QF, et al. A long noncoding RNA activated by TGF-beta promotes the invasion-metastasis cascade in hepatocellular carcinoma. Cancer Cell. 2014;**25**:666-681. DOI: 10.1016/j.ccr.2014.03.010

[212] Han F, Wang C, Wang Y, Zhang L. Long noncoding RNA ATB promotes osteosarcoma cell proliferation, migration and invasion by suppressing miR-200s. American Journal of Cancer Research. 2017;**7**(4):770-783

[213] Chaturvedi MM, Sung B, Yadav VR, Kannappan R, Aggarwal BB. NF-κB addiction and its role in cancer: 'One size does not fit all'. Oncogene. 2010;**30**(14):1615-1630. DOI: 10.1038/onc.2010.566

[214] Bird L. lncRNA NKILA: A killer regulator. Nature Reviews. Immunology. 2018;**18**(11):666-667. DOI: 10.1038/s41577-018-0078-3

[215] Liu B, Sun L, Liu Q, Gong C, Yao Y, Lv X, et al. A cytoplasmic NF-κB interacting long noncoding RNA blocks IκB phosphorylation and suppresses breast cancer metastasis. Cancer Cell. 2015;**27**(3):370-381. DOI: 10.1016/j.ccell.2015.02.004

[216] Li X, Shen JK, Hornicek FJ, Xiao T, Duan Z. Noncoding RNA in drug resistant sarcoma. Oncotarget. 2017; **8**(40):69086-69104. DOI: 10.18632/oncotarget.19029

[217] Zhu KP, Ma XL, Zhang CL. LncRNA ODRUL contributes to osteosarcoma progression through the miR-3182/MMP2 axis. Molecular Therapy. 2017;**25**(10):2383-2393. DOI: 10.1016/j.ymthe.2017.06.027

[218] Wang Y, Huang Y, Xiang P, Tian W. LncRNA expression and implication in osteosarcoma: A systematic review and meta-analysis. OncoTargets and Therapy. 2017;**10**:5355-5361. DOI: 10.2147/OTT.S149889

[219] Kong D, Wang Y. Knockdown of lncRNA HULC inhibits proliferation, migration, invasion, and promotes apoptosis by sponging miR-122 in osteosarcoma. Journal of Cellular Biochemistry. 2018 Jan;**119**(1): 1050-1061. DOI: 10.1002/jcb.26273

[220] Cui X, Jing X, Long C, Tian J, Zhu J. Long noncoding RNA MEG3, a potential novel biomarker to predict the clinical outcome of cancer patients: A meta-analysis. Oncotarget. 2017;**8**(12): 19049-19056. DOI: 10.18632/oncotarget.14987

[221] Sun L, Yang C, Xu J, Feng Y, Wang L, Cui T. Long noncoding RNA EWSAT1 promotes osteosarcoma cell growth and metastasis through suppression of MEG3 expression. DNA and Cell Biology. 2016;**35**(12):812-818. DOI: 10.1089/dna.2016.3467

[222] An N, Cheng D. The long noncoding RNA HOST2 promotes gemcitabine resistance in human pancreatic cancer cells. Pathology and Oncology Research. 2018;**24**:1-7. DOI: 10.1007/s12253-018-0486-5.

[223] Huang FX, Chen HJ, Zheng FX, Gao ZY, Sun PF, Peng Q, et al. LncRNA BLACAT1 is involved in chemoresistance of non-small cell lung cancer cells by regulating autophagy. International Journal of Oncology. 2018; **54**(1):339-347. DOI: 10.3892/ijo.2018.4614

[224] Zhu QN, Wang G, Guo Y, et al. LncRNA H19 is a major mediator of doxorubicin chemoresistance in breast cancer cells through a cullin4A-MDR1 pathway. Oncotarget. 2017;**8**(54): 91990-92003. DOI: 10.18632/oncotarget.21121

[225] Chen X, Xie R, Gu P, Huang M, Han J, Dong W, et al. Long noncoding RNA LBCS inhibits self-renewal and chemoresistance of bladder cancer stem cells through epigenetic silencing of SOX2. Clinical Cancer Research. 2018. pii: clincanres.1656.2018. DOI: 10.1158/1078-0432.CCR-18-1656

[226] Wang H, Liu M, Fang L, et al. The cisplatin-induced lncRNA PANDAR dictates the chemoresistance of ovarian cancer via regulating SFRS2-mediated p53 phosphorylation. Cell Death & Disease. 2018;**9**(11):1103. Published 2018 Oct 30. DOI: 10.1038/s41419-018-1148-y

[227] Ding B, Lou W, Xu L, Fan W. Non-coding RNA in drug resistance of hepatocellular carcinoma. Bioscience Reports. 2018;**38**(5):BSR20180915. DOI: 10.1042/BSR20180915

[228] He H, Ni J, Huang J. Molecular mechanisms of chemoresistance in osteosarcoma (Review). Oncology Letters. 2014;7(5):1352-1362. DOI: 10.3892/ol.2014.1935

[229] Kun-Peng Z, Xiao-Long M, Chun-Lin Z. LncRNA FENDRR sensitizes doxorubicin-resistance of osteosarcoma cells through down-regulating ABCB1 and ABCC1. Oncotarget. 2017;**8**(42): 71881-71893. DOI: 10.18632/oncotarget.17985

[230] Zhang CL, Zhu KP, Ma XL. Antisense lncRNA FOXC2-AS1 promotes doxorubicin resistance in osteosarcoma by increasing the expression of FOXC2. Cancer Letters. 2017;**396**:66-75. DOI: 10.1016/j.canlet.2017.03.018

[231] Li Z, Zhao L, Wang Q. Overexpression of long non-coding RNA HOTTIP increases chemoresistance of osteosarcoma cell by activating the Wnt/β-catenin pathway. American Journal of Translational Research. 2016;**8**(5):2385-2393

[232] Wang Y, Zhang L, Zheng X, Zhong W, Tian X, Yin B, et al. Long non-coding RNA LINC00161 sensitises osteosarcoma cells to cisplatin-induced apoptosis by regulating the miR-645-IFIT2 axis. Cancer Letters. 2016;**382**(2):137-146. DOI: 10.1016/j.canlet.2016.08.024

[233] Zhang Y, Yang J, Zhao N, et al. Progress in the chemotherapeutic treatment of osteosarcoma. Oncology Letters. 2018;**16**(5):6228-6237. DOI: 10.3892/ol.2018.9434

[234] Hegyi M, Arany A, Semsei AF, et al. Pharmacogenetic analysis of high-dose methotrexate treatment in children with osteosarcoma. Oncotarget. 2016;**8**(6):9388-9398. DOI: 10.18632/oncotarget.11543

[235] Han Z, Shi L. Long non-coding RNA LUCAT1 modulates methotrexate resistance in osteosarcoma via miR-200c/ABCB1 axis. Biochemical and Biophysical Research Communications. 2018;**495**(1):947-953. DOI: 10.1016/j.bbrc.2017.11.121

[236] Zhu KP, Zhang CL, Shen GQ, Zhu ZS. Long noncoding RNA expression profiles of the doxorubicin-resistant human osteosarcoma cell line MG63/DXR and its parental cell line MG63 as ascertained by microarray analysis. International Journal of Clinical and Experimental Pathology. 2015;**8**(8):8754-8773

[237] Zhang CL, Zhu KP, Shen GQ, Zhu ZS. A long non-coding RNA contributes to doxorubicin resistance of osteosarcoma. Tumour Biology. 2016;**37**(2):2737-2748. DOI: 10.1007/s13277-015-4130-7

[238] Slaby O, Laga R, Sedlacek O. Therapeutic targeting of non-coding RNAs in cancer. The Biochemical Journal. 2017 Dec 14;**474**(24):4219-4251. DOI: 10.1042/BCJ20170079

[239] Ling H, Fabbri M, Calin GA. MicroRNAs and other non-coding RNAs as targets for anticancer drug development. Nature Reviews. Drug Discovery. 2013;**12**(11):847-865. DOI: 10.1038/nrd4140

[240] Lavorgna G, Vago R, Sarmini M, Montorsi F, Salonia A, Bellone M. Long non-coding RNAs as novel therapeutic targets in cancer. Pharmacological Research. 2016;**110**:131-138. DOI: 10.1016/j.phrs.2016.05.018

[241] Palmieri G, Paliogiannis P, Sini MC, Manca A, Palomba G, Doneddu V, et al. Long non-coding RNA CASC2 in human cancer. Critical Reviews in Oncology/Hematology. 2017;**111**:31-38. DOI: 10.1016/j.critrevonc.2017.01.003

[242] Ba Z, Gu L, Hao S, Wang X, Cheng Z, Nie G. Downregulation of lncRNA CASC2 facilitates osteosarcoma growth and invasion through miR-181a. Cell Proliferation. 2018;**51**(1):e12409. DOI: 10.1111/cpr.12409

[243] Wang Y, Kong D. LncRNA GAS5 represses osteosarcoma cells growth and metastasis via sponging MiR-203a. Cellular Physiology and Biochemistry. 2018;**45**(2):844-855. DOI: 10.1159/000487178

[244] Ye K, Wang S, Zhang H, Han H, Ma B, Nan W. Long noncoding RNA GAS5 suppresses cell growth and epithelial-mesenchymal transition in osteosarcoma by regulating the miR-221/ARHI pathway. Journal of Cellular Biochemistry. 2017;**118**(12):4772-4781. DOI: 10.1002/jcb.26145

[245] Kirschmann DA, Seftor EA, Hardy KM, Seftor RE, Hendrix MJ. Molecular pathways: Vasculogenic mimicry in tumor cells: Diagnostic and therapeutic implications. Clinical Cancer Research. 2012;**18**:2726-2732. DOI: 10.1158/1078-0432.CCR-11-3237

[246] Zhang Y, Dai Q, Zeng F, Liu H. MALAT1 promotes the proliferation and metastasis of osteosarcoma cells by activating the RAC1/JNK pathway via targeting miR-509. Oncology Research. 2018;**26**:1-32. DOI: 10.3727/096504017X14957939026111

[247] Liu K, Huang J, Ni J, Song D, Ding M, Wang J, et al. MALAT1 promotes osteosarcoma development by regulation of HMGB1 via miR-142-3p and miR-129-5p. Cell Cycle. 2017;**16**: 578-587. DOI: 10.1080/15384101.2017.1288324

[248] Yang C, Wang G, Yang J, Wang L. Long noncoding RNA NBAT1 negatively modulates growth and metastasis of osteosarcoma cells through suppression of miR-21. American Journal of Cancer Research. 2017;7: 2009-2019

[249] Kotake Y, Goto T, Naemura M, Inoue Y, Okamoto H, Tahara K. Long noncoding RNA PANDA positively regulates proliferation of osteosarcoma cells. Anticancer Research. 2017;**37**:81-85. DOI: 10.21873/anticanres.11292

[250] Zou Y, Zhong Y, Wu J, Xiao H, Zhang X, Liao X, et al. Long non-coding PANDAR as a novel biomarker in human cancer: A systematic review. Cell Proliferation. 2018;**51**(1):e12422. DOI: 10.1111/cpr.12422

[251] Zhou Q, Chen F, Zhao J, Li B, Liang Y, Pan W, et al. Long non-coding RNA PVT1 promotes osteosarcoma development by acting as a molecular sponge to regulate miR-195. Oncotarget. 2016;**7**(50):82620-82633. DOI: 10.18632/oncotarget.13012

[252] Song J, Wu X, Liu F, Li M, Sun Y, Wang Y, et al. Long non-coding RNA PVT1 promotes glycolysis and tumor progression by regulating miR-497/HK2 axis in osteosarcoma. Biochemical and Biophysical Research Communications. 2017;**490**(2):217-224. DOI: 10.1016/j.bbrc.2017.06.024

[253] Chen X, Zhou Y, Liu S, Zhang D, Yang X, Zhou Q, et al. LncRNA TP73-AS1 predicts poor prognosis and functions as oncogenic lncRNA in osteosarcoma. Journal of Cellular Biochemistry. 2018;**120**(2):2569-2575. DOI: 10.1002/jcb.27556

[254] Yang G, Song R, Wang L, Wu X. Knockdown of long non-coding RNA TP73-AS1 inhibits osteosarcoma cell proliferation and invasion through sponging miR-142. Biomedicine & Pharmacotherapy. 2018;**103**:1238-1245. DOI: 10.1016/j.biopha.2018.04.146

[255] Bonnetti A, Carninci P. From bench to bedside: The long journey of long non-coding RNAs. Current Opinion in Systems Biology. 2017;**33**:119-124. DOI: https://doi.org/10.1016/j.coisb.2017.04.016

[256] Adams BD, Parsons C, Walker L, Zhang WC, Slack FJ. Targeting noncoding RNAs in disease. The Journal of Clinical Investigation. 2017;**127**(3): 761-771. DOI: 10.1172/JCI84424

[257] Fatemi RP, Velmeshev D, Faghihi MA. De-repressing LncRNA-targeted genes to upregulate gene expression: Focus on small molecule therapeutics.

Molecular Therapy–Nucleic Acids. 2014;**3**(11):e196. DOI: 10.1038/mtna.2014.45

[258] Raimondi L, De Luca A, Costa V, et al. Circulating biomarkers in osteosarcoma: New translational tools for diagnosis and treatment. Oncotarget. 2017;**8**(59):100831-100851. DOI: 10.18632/oncotarget.19852

Chapter 4

A Novel Strategy of Dual Inhibition of Distinct Metabolic Features in Osteosarcoma

Shingo Kishi, Kanya Honoki, Yasuhito Tanaka and Hiroki Kuniyasu

Abstract

Mitochondria are the places for the energy production of the cells, while reactive oxygen species (ROS) are also produced alongside. In recent years, it has been reported that cancer stem cells metabolize predominantly through oxidative phosphorylation (OXPHOS) rather than glycolysis. Targeting OXPHOS achieved by suppression of ATP synthesis through mitochondrial ATP synthase could be a potential therapeutic option against cancer stem cells. Since c-Myc inhibition is considered to lead a metabolic flux to OXPHOS from glycolysis, the combinatory inhibition of both OXPHOS and glycolysis could be a strong candidate for the treatment of malignant tumors. In this chapter, we will discuss about the mitochondria metabolism as the potential therapeutic target in osteosarcoma stem cells, and the synergistic effects of combination of OXPHOS inhibitor with c-Myc inhibitor, which target both OXPHOS-dominant cancer stem cells and glycolysis-dominant non-cancer stem cells, will be discussed.

Keywords: osteosarcoma, mitochondria, metabolism, OXPHOS, c-Myc

1. Introduction

Intratumor heterogeneity, which is the basis of tumor evolution, is the fundamental challenge in cancer medicine. Intratumor heterogeneity is considered to be involved in several important aspects in cancer biology such as disease relapse and metastatic behaviors as well as drug resistance. Over the past decades, a small subset of tumor cells, so-called cancer stem cells (CSCs), have been proposed to be a hierarchical organizer of the tumor heterogeneity [1] and play a critical role in tumor relapse, metastasis, drug resistance, and tumor propagation in many cancer types including osteosarcoma (OS) [2–6]. At the apex of the heterogeneity in the tumor, CSCs possess the capacity of self-renew and tumorigenicity which generate the bulk of tumor with more differentiated progenies [7]. Conventional anticancer therapies target the bulk of heterogeneous tumor mass resulting in tumor shrinkage, but CSCs could trigger the relapse by differentiation into non-stem tumor cells. Thus, targeting CSCs could represent an integral component for developing more effective treatment strategies against cancer.

Now, we have evidences that cancer heterogeneity not only is generated by genetically distinct subclones but is also driven by phenotypic and functional

IntechOpen

heterogeneity within each subclone [8, 9]. One of the distinct phenotypes of CSCs is their cellular metabolism mechanisms for energy production. Tumor cells reprogram their metabolic machinery to meet their needs during tumor growth known as Warburg effect which shifts their ATP production from via oxidative phosphorylation (OXPHOS) to glycolysis even in the microenvironment with abundant oxygen concentration [10]. Over the past years, the metabolic phenotype of CSCs has been intensely investigated, and it was originally hypothesized that CSCs would reflect the normal tissue hierarchy where multipotent stem cells are fundamentally glycolytic, while differentiated somatic cells rely on OXPHOS [11]. Although the differentiated cells increase their dependency upon the glycolysis during the acquisition of the transformed phenotype, these changes might be cell specific, and some cells might adapt to neoplastic transformation by increasing their dependency on OXPHOS [12]. As a matter of fact, the metabolic phenotype of CSCs are controversial suggesting that it could be a tumor-type- or cell line-dependent manner such as breast and nasopharyngeal CSCs relying on glycolysis [13, 14], while lung, glioblastoma and pancreatic ductal adenocarcinoma CSCs relying on OXSPHOS [15–17]. In osteosarcoma (OS), a CSC-like cell line, 3AB-OS, exhibited its metabolic dependency on glycolysis compared to the parental MG-63 cells [18]. However, this came from only one cell line chemically treated long time from MG-63 which bore the *ras* gene mutation unusually found in OS. Controversially, there is the evidence that the transformed mesenchymal stem cells (MSCs), which are supposed to be the sarcoma-initiating cells or sarcoma stem cells, showed the increased OXPHOS and had a capability to switch to glycolysis to adapt to their microenvironments [19]. The discrepancy in these metabolic profiles of CSCs would be due to multifactorial causes. The first possible explanation is the plasticity of these cells in response to the microenvironment and the stages of harvesting in terms of differentiation/dedifferentiation [20]. Another possible cause would be the lack of precise definition of CSCs and their heterogeneity due to the various techniques for CSC isolation [21]. Furthermore, the metabolic status of CSCs can be affected by cross talk between CSCs and cancer-associated stroma in the microenvironment. For instance, OS cells directly increase their mitochondrial biogenesis using this energy-rich metabolite such as lactate that is abundantly provided by MSC as an effect of the altered microenvironmental conditions induced by OS cells, and the lactate produced by MSC promotes the migratory ability of OS cell [22].

Actually, there are several reports indicating that CSCs have augmented utilization of extracellular catabolites such as pyruvate, lactate to support OXPHOS, [23] and mitochondrial metabolism could be a potential target for an effective elimination of CSCs [17]. Previous studies suggested that inhibition of the OXPHOS pathway reduced sphere formation and tumor formation capacity, which demonstrated the vulnerability of CSCs to mitochondria-targeted therapies [24], and several agents such as salinomycin targeting CSCs through inhibition of mitochondrial biogenesis and OXPHOS are currently under investigation for cancer treatment [25].

Here, we will discuss about the mitochondrial metabolism as a potential therapeutic target in osteosarcoma, especially its stem-like cell populations.

2. Myc is a key regulator of cancer cell metabolism

Glucose is one of the major nutrients that mammalian cells utilize to synthesize new organelles as well as to generate high-energy molecules, such as ATP, NADH/NADPH, and FADH. c-Myc played an important role in regulation of glycolysis through its target glucose metabolism genes [26], and those genes directly regulated by c-Myc include glucose transporter GLUT1, hexokinase 2

(HK2), phosphofructokinase (PFKM), and enolase 1 (ENO1) [27, 28]. Myc was also observed to upregulate lactate dehydrogenase A (LDHA) to generate NAD+, which is a cofactor required for the glycolysis particularly by GAPDH [29]. Through the upregulation of these genes, c-Myc contributes directly to the Warburg effect (aerobic glycolysis) and the ability of transformed cells to convert glucose to pyruvate even under adequate oxygen tension. Myc also regulates protein synthesis, ribosome biogenesis, nucleotide biosynthesis, as well as fatty acid and cholesterol metabolism. Cancer cells take advantage of these Myc's broad reaches to reprogram and augment the most critical processes for survival, particularly metabolism.

In addition to the metabolic reprogramming, c-Myc also contributes to the cell cycle regulation in corporation with PI3K (phosphatidylinositol-3,4,5-triphosphate)/Akt/mTOR (mammalian target of rapamycin) and Wnt pathway. The role of PI3K-Akt-mTOR and Wnt pathways in regulation of the cell cycle progression in cancer cell has been proposed (**Figure 1**). The activation of insulin/insulin-like growth factor (IGF) receptor by nutrients/growth factors activates PI3K-Akt pathway. The phosphorylated Akt activates mammalian target of rapamycin complex 1 (mTORC1), and the activated mTORC1 upregulates the protein synthesis but inhibits autophagy. Inhibition of autophagy rescues Dvl (Dish homolog in mammalian), and this leads to activation of Wnt pathway. Wnt pathway is the key pathway in activation of cell cycle, and the activated Wnt pathway upregulates the CyclinD; the c-Myc; the matrix metalloproteinases, COX-2, peroxisome proliferator-activated receptors (PPARs); and the growth factors and their receptors and downregulates E-cadherin, the cell cycle inhibitor p16INK4a (ARF), and p53 [30]. Wnt pathway thus regulates the cancer cell entry into the cell cycle through the production of

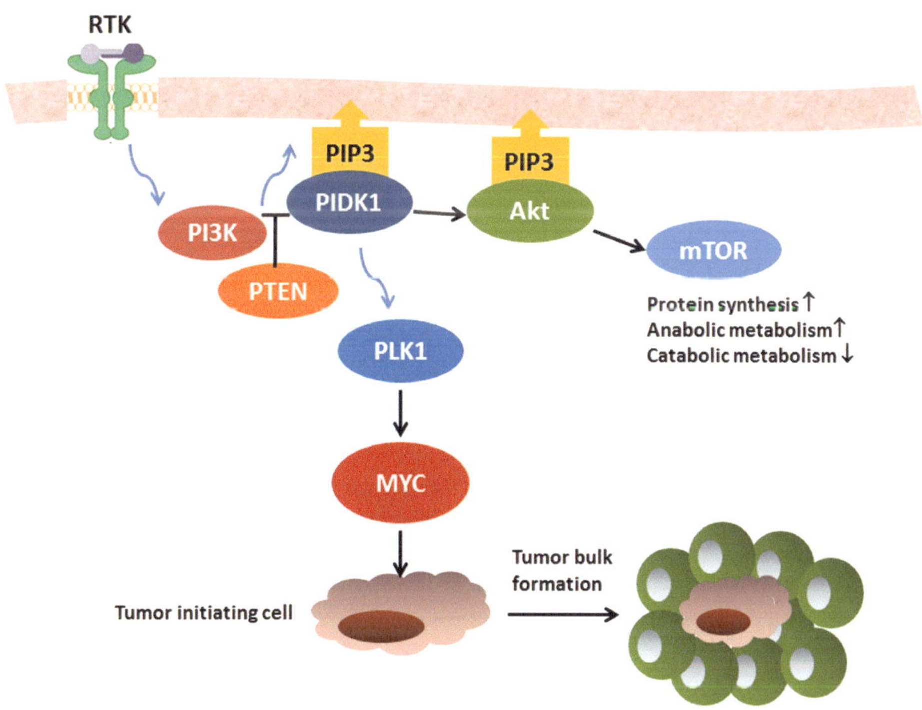

Figure 1.
c-Myc contributes to the cell cycle regulation in corporation with PI3K/Akt/mTOR and Wnt pathway. The activation of insulin/IGF receptor by nutrients/growth factors activates PI3K-Akt pathway. The phosphorylated Akt activates mTORC1, which eventually leads to activation of Wnt pathway. Wnt pathway is the key pathway in activation of cell cycle, and the activated Wnt pathway upregulates the CyclinD, the c-Myc which would be involved in tumor initiation as well as tumor progression.

CyclinD. CyclinD complexes with cyclin-dependent kinase 4/6 (Cdk4/6), inactivates the tumor suppressor protein retinoblastoma (Rb), and promotes the entry of the cell from G0 to G1 phase of cell cycle as well as metabolic reprogramming through the c-Myc activation as described above. In this context, c-Myc is acknowledged to play an important role to activate genes involved in predominantly cell cycle regulation, cellular metabolism, and protein synthesis, especially specific to G0-G-S transition as well as glycolysis and Krebs cycle, chromatin structure, and its transcriptional networks in cancer cells and embryonic stem cells as well [31, 32]. Given its crucial role in cancer progression and maintenance, c-Myc has been the ideal target for cancer therapy, and c-Myc targeting strategy in cancer therapy has been investigated in various means such as direct inhibition by antisense oligonucleotide [33] and siRNA [34], indirect inhibition by blocking transcription with BET bromodomain inhibitors such as JQ-1 [35], and blocking mRNA translation with mTOR inhibitor [36]. After a long time struggling on targeting c-Myc in cancer therapy, we are now witnessing a renewed interest in making Myc inhibition for the future cancer therapy. In the aspect of c-Myc contribution to the metabolism, c-Myc promotes a Warburg-like glycolytic phenotype through dual mechanism of upregulation of key glycolytic enzymes as described above, and suppression of peroxisome proliferator-activated receptor gamma coactivator 1-alpha (PGC-1α) by direct inhibition through binding to its promoter [17]. PGC-1α is crucial for the anti-oxidative capacity and mitochondrial metabolism in cancer [37, 38] and contributes to the maintenance of CSC's phenotype of self-renewal through controlling intracellular ROS levels. Myc/PGC-1α balance controls the metabolic phenotype of cancer cells as c-Myc dominance shifts to Warburg phenotype of differentiated cancer cells and PGC-1α dominance shifts to OXPHOS-dependent phenotype of CSCs [17]. Therefore, combining OXPHOS inhibition with c-Myc inhibition could provide a new multimodal approach for targeting the distinct metabolic features in cancer therapy.

3. Cancer stem cell metabolism: a potential therapeutic target

CSCs also known as tumor-initiating cells (TICs) are a rare population of tumor cells with stem cell properties, which are thought to generate the tumor bulk and considered to drive the malignant growth, treatment resistance, minimal residual disease, and metastases. Along with the role of cancer drivers, CSCs also exhibit stem cell properties such as self-renewal and multilineage differentiation capacity [39]. CSCs are considered to be resistant to chemotherapy or radiations, both of which successfully destroy differentiated non stem-like cancer cells. As a matter of fact, even though current conventional anticancer therapies could achieve a transient control over the disease, a large number of patients experience tumor relapse or metastatic dissemination after an initial treatment with apparent disease-free period. Since CSCs, resisting to conventional therapies, attributes these biological behaviors, eradication of CSCs could be a promising target to totally exterminate the disease of cancer [40].

Although much is known regarding metabolic pathways important for cancer cell survival, the potential for therapeutic metabolic alteration of CSCs has not been fully uncovered [41], but recent studies indicate that metabolism and stemness are highly intertwined processes in tumor tissues, and CSCs possibly have different metabolic properties compared to non-CSCs.

Glucose homeostasis is reciprocally controlled by the catabolic glycolysis/OXPHOS and by the anabolic gluconeogenesis pathway. In the catabolic reaction, when oxygen is absent, glycolysis predominantly controls the metabolism of ATP production, while in the presence of oxygen, OXPHOS predominantly regulates the maximal ATP production in the mitochondria. Cancer cells preferentially metabolize glucose rather than OXPHOS even in the presence of oxygen defined as Warburg effect/aerobic glycolysis by the activation of some key genes such as c-Myc. In contrast to the somatic cells which primarily utilize OXPHOS, pluripotent stem cells including embryonal stem cells and induced pluripotent stem cells rely on glycolysis [42]. Therefore, it has to be pointed out that the biological functions of CSCs are different from those of differentiated cancer cells, making their phenotype more similar to normal stem cell, and metabolism is not the exception. Since aerobic glycolysis/Warburg effect has been widely accepted and recognized as a peculiar hallmark of cancer cells, it may be reasonable to expect that, conversely, CSC metabolism is mostly oriented toward mitochondrial OXPHOS. Actually, it is broadly accepted that ATP production in CSCs depends on glycolysis or OXPHOS in a tumor-type-dependent manner. The heterogeneity and plasticity of CSCs probably determine their primary source of energy to survive. The recent investigation has suggested that CSCs may display a broader repertoire of biochemical behavior in response to different environmental conditions, and accumulating evidence has indicated that CSCs utilize OXPHOS not only relying on the glycolysis [41, 43]. CSC metabolism show a highly plastic profile which allows to fulfill the energy requirements, according to the most suitable environmental condition. This metabolic flexibility of CSCs has been shown in diverse tumor types demonstrating that CSCs efficiently gain energy production from glycolysis when OXPHOS is blocked [44]. Recently, De Francesco et al. proposed the "two metabolic hit strategies" for eradication of CSCs (**Figure 2**) [45]. They demonstrated that the prolonged treatment with a mitochondria-interfering agent like doxycycline drastically impairs oxygen consumption rate (OCR) and mitochondrial respiration in MCF7 breast cancer cells. Such impairment in mitochondrial activity represents a first metabolic hit that constrains cellular metabolism of the surviving cancer cell subpopulation toward a

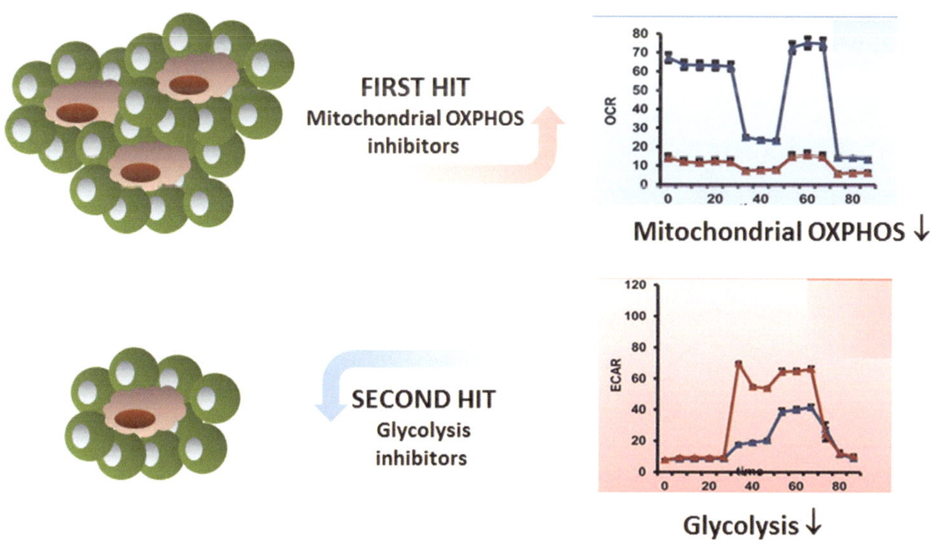

Figure 2.
The treatment with a mitochondria-interfering agent impairs oxygen consumption rate (OCR) and mitochondrial respiration in cancer cells as a metabolic first hit that constrains cellular metabolism of the surviving cancer cell subpopulation toward a predominantly glycolytic phenotype, resulting in metabolic inflexibility, as evidenced by the increased extracellular acidification rate (ECAR). The use of a glycolysis inhibitor may therefore act as the second metabolic hit that efficiently targets CSCs by halting their biochemical machinery (X axis, time (min); Y axis, pmoles/min/mg protein; red line, mitochondria inhibitor treatment; blue line, control).

predominantly glycolytic phenotype, resulting in metabolic inflexibility, as evidenced by the increased extracellular acidification rate (ECAR). In this sequence, the glycolysis inhibitor potentially acts a second metabolic hit which effectively targets CSCs. Thus, specific metabolic-oriented pharmacological intervention could reverse CSC metabolic plasticity toward an inflexible biochemical phenotype, representing a new synthetic-lethal metabolic strategy for eradicating CSCs.

4. Targeting mitochondrial physiology in cancer stem cells

Mitochondria are key organelles involved in several processes related to cell proliferation and survival, and their most important function is the generation of ATP which holds cell metabolism. As the main energy producers, mitochondria produce ATP using tricarboxylic acid (TCA) cycle and OXPHOS. They also generate reactive oxygen species (ROS) during this process, which are sometimes harmful to the cells when produced excessively.

Because mitochondria play a key role in the alteration of oxidative stress and energy status, their functional characteristics have been considered to verify stemness like stem cell stability and pluripotency [46, 47]. Mitochondrial metabolic activity and antioxidant enzyme expression have shown to be closely related to the cell differentiation [48, 49]. Thus, we could assume that stem cell mitochondria play important roles in maintaining stemness and differentiation. However, whether the roles of CSC mitochondria are similar to stem cell mitochondria or so-called differentiated cancer cells in general is not clear. Based on the previous reports, the CSCs might be more differentiated than normal stem cells, and the mitochondrial properties of CSCs are possibly different from those of stem cells or general cancer cells [39, 50].

Mitochondria have a multi-level network of antioxidant and OXPHOS systems (**Figure 3**). Mitochondrial redox balances are regulated by the mitochondrial inner membrane electrochemical gradient. As shown in **Figure 3**, nicotinamide adenine dinucleotide (NADH) from TCA cycle is oxidized by Complex I in the electron transport chain (ETC) of OXPHOS. Electrons from Complex I and II are

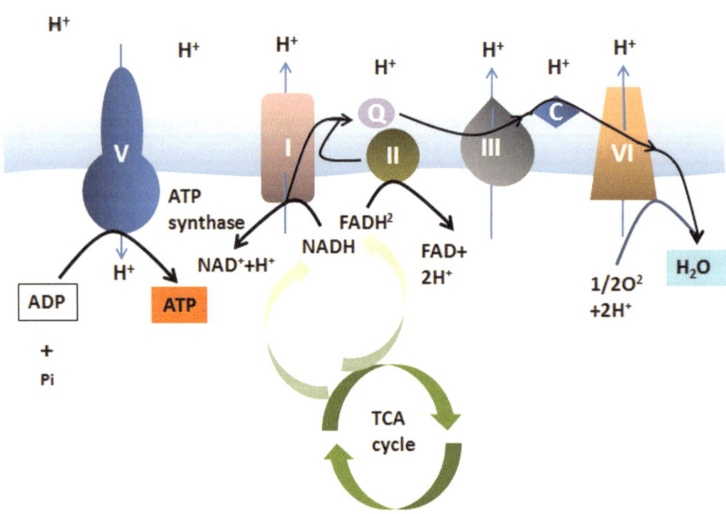

Figure 3.
Mitochondrial redox balances are regulated by the mitochondrial inner membrane electrochemical gradient. NADH from TCA cycle is oxidized by Complex I in the ETC. Electrons from Complex I and II are transferred to coenzyme Q10 and then passed on to Complex III, cytochrome c, Complex IV, and finally O_2 to generate H_2O. Complex V (FoF1-ATP synthase) generates ATP from ADP for the cellular energy source.

transferred to coenzyme Q10 and then passed on to Complex III, cytochrome c, Complex IV, and finally O_2 to generate H_2O. Complex V (ATP synthase; F0-F1) generates ATP from ADP as well as inorganic phosphate Pi.

A powerful strategy focused on mitochondrial biogenetics as a target to eradicate CSCs involves inhibition of the ETC complex, with consequent ROS overproduction. Dong et al. demonstrated that the suppression of mitochondrial Complex I activity inhibited oxygen consumption and induced glycolysis in breast CSCs as a result of loss of fructose-1,6-biphosphatase implying that overproduction of ROS and reduction in glucose metabolism might be effective against breast CSCs [11]. Hirsch et al. also showed that metformin, the first-line antidiabetic drug, selectively killed the CSCs in breast cancer cell line through the inhibition of Complex I [51]. Furthermore, atovaquone, an FDA-approved antimalarial drug, inhibits the propagation of breast cancer cell line MCF7-derived CSCs through the selective OXPHOS inhibition by targeting the CoQ10 dependence of mitochondrial Complex III [52]. This has been explored in the context of therapy as indicated by Alvero et al. using the novel isoflavone derivative NV-128 which significantly decreased mitochondrial function, as shown by a decrease in ATP, Complex I and Complex IV levels, and induced cell death in ovarian CSCs [53]. Finally, mitochondria-targeted vitamin E succinate (MitoVES) has been well characterized as an agent, which potentiates the ability to induce apoptosis in breast CSCs [54]. Reduction of mitochondrial membrane potential, overproduction of mitochondrial ROS, and inhibition of mitochondrial biogenesis have been demonstrated to affect CSC proliferation and survival [55]. These inputs indicate that the maintenance of CSC proliferation may not only be dependent on glycolysis, but is also based on mitochondrial activity. Therefore, the specific mitochondrial-targeted compounds which induce cell death in chemoresistant CSCs are promising novel therapeutic venue to treat cancer patients with relapsed or metastatic diseases. The most important point is that mitochondria from CSCs are not indistinguishable to those from differentiated non stem-like tumor cells in divergent aspects. Since CSCs are considered to be heterogeneous and adaptive metabolic profiles, the future therapy targeting cellular metabolism should be designed in a form of simultaneous or selective blockade of both glycolysis and mitochondrial respiration to completely eradicate CSCs [20]. Consequently, dual inhibition of glycolytic and mitochondrial energy pathways has proven to be effective against tumor growth in a number of preclinical cancer models. For instance, dual inhibition of glycolysis by 2-deoxyglucose (2-DG) and OXPHOS by metformin is effective in vivo against breast cancer cell xenograft model [56]. However, hexokinase inhibitors such as 2-DG and 3-bromopyruvate have been unfortunately discontinued in clinical trials. There has been an elegant study demonstrating sarcoma cells to be more sensitive than normal cells to dual inhibition of glycolysis with 2-deoxyglucose and OXPHOS with oligomycin or metformin [57]. Recently, Kang et al. have demonstrated that ALDH inhibitor gossypol combined with mitochondrial Complex I inhibitor phenformin resulted in up to 80% ATP depletion in non-small cell lung cancer, which induced significant tumor regression in the cancer xenograft model [58]. These warrant that a key molecule regulating cancer energy metabolism can be a therapeutic target.

Meanwhile, other mitochondria-related processes like activation of developmental signaling pathways including Hedgehog, Notch, and Wnt are also the druggable targets; the drug targeting Notch and Hedgehog pathway has been developed [59], and numerous molecules acting on mitochondria has been used or being tested in clinical trials [60]. Adding these attempts targeting mitochondria, we will emphasize that the dual inhibition of metabolic pathways could be an approach with greater potential to eradicate heterogeneous CSCs rather than singularly targeting glycolysis or OXPHOS pathway.

5. Novel approach to target cellular metabolism in osteosarcoma

Osteosarcoma and mitochondria have been investigated since 1970; however, those are mostly limited to the morphological characteristics by microscopic or electron microscopic observation [61, 62].

Giang et al. demonstrated that highly invasive and metastatic cell lines were more relied on Warburg effect-like glycolysis than their parental cell lines which showed similar mitochondrial oxygen consumption rate to fetal osteoblasts, suggesting that highly metastatic and invasive cell lines were in the state of suppression of mitochondrial function and upregulation of glycolysis. They suggested that the mechanism of mitochondrial dysfunction was the results of mitochondrial permeability transition such as mitochondrial swelling, depolarization, and membrane permeabilization, and they also demonstrated that this mitochondrial dysfunction and the Warburg effect are reversed by the treatment with mitochondrial permeability transition inhibitor sanglifehrin A [63]. These results indicated that osteosarcoma cells might possess the metabolic plasticity in response to their microenvironment especially hypoxia-reoxygenation caused by an irregular blood supply within tumors, an immature and leaky vasculature, and an abnormal and constantly changing vessel network architecture.

Another biochemical mechanism which contributes to the glycolytic rate of tumor cells is the inhibition of mitochondrial ATP synthase (F1F0-ATPase) by the natural inhibitor protein IF_1 [64]. Barbato et al. reported that IF_1 modulates the mitochondrial membrane potential and oxidative phosphorylation rate in osteosarcoma cells suggesting that interaction between IF_1 and FoF1-ATPase might regulate the OXPHOS and glycolysis [65]. However, the detailed mechanisms regulating the cellular bioenergetics by IF_1 have been still controversial in cancer cells under the complex microenvironment.

Recently, novel strategy targeting CSCs through phytochemicals and their analogs has been proposed, and mitochondria are one of their potential targets [66]. Among the various compounds, pterostilbene (PTE), which is a methylated resveratrol derived from plants, has been shown to inhibit CSC properties in breast cancer [67, 68], glioma [69], hepatocellular carcinoma [70], and lung cancer [71] through the inhibition of multiple pathways which are possibly related to the CSC propagation such as Wnt, Hedgehog, Notch, and PI3K/Akt. Honokiol (HNK), which is the extract from *Magnolia obovata*, has shown its various antitumor effects through the inhibition of several pathways such as PI3K/Akt/mTOR, Wnt, and c-Myc [72–74]. Besides these effects of PTE and HNK, we have identified that PTE in combination with HNK could be the possible metabolism-targeted therapy against osteosarcoma as a "two hit" or "dual inhibition" of metabolic pathways, OXPHOS and glycolysis. PTE treatment on human osteosarcoma cell lines SaOS2, U2OS, and MG63 reduced viabilities of all cell lines in dose-dependent manner, and expression of stem cell marker such as Oct3, NS, and CD44 and the ability of sphere formation were also decreased in terms of sphere number and size (**Figure 4a**). PTE reduced the activity of F0F1-ATP synthase, Complex V predominantly (**Figure 4b**), and the mitochondrial oxygen consumption rates and synthetic amount of ATP were also decreased in spheroid condition (**Figure 4c**). These results suggest that PTE possibly targets stem cell population which preferably relies on OXPHOS, suppressing ATP synthesis via F0F1-ATP synthase inhibition as well as increased ROS production in osteosarcoma cells, and changes metabolic flax to glycolysis-dependent feature.

As aforementioned before, c-Myc promotes a Warburg-like glycolytic phenotype through the upregulation of key glycolytic enzymes along with the suppression of PGC-1α. There are several reports regarding the anticancer activity of HNK which is possibly associated with c-Myc as well as JQ1, a BET bromodomain inhibitor [74]. Thus, we conducted dual inhibition of OXPHOS by PTE and c-Myc inhibition by HNK or JQ1. The results showed that both of these agents synergistically inhibited osteosarcoma cell growth in a dose-dependent manner (**Figure 5**). Now, we are conducting an investigation of dual metabolic inhibition via in vivo experiments using our own established rat osteosarcoma model.

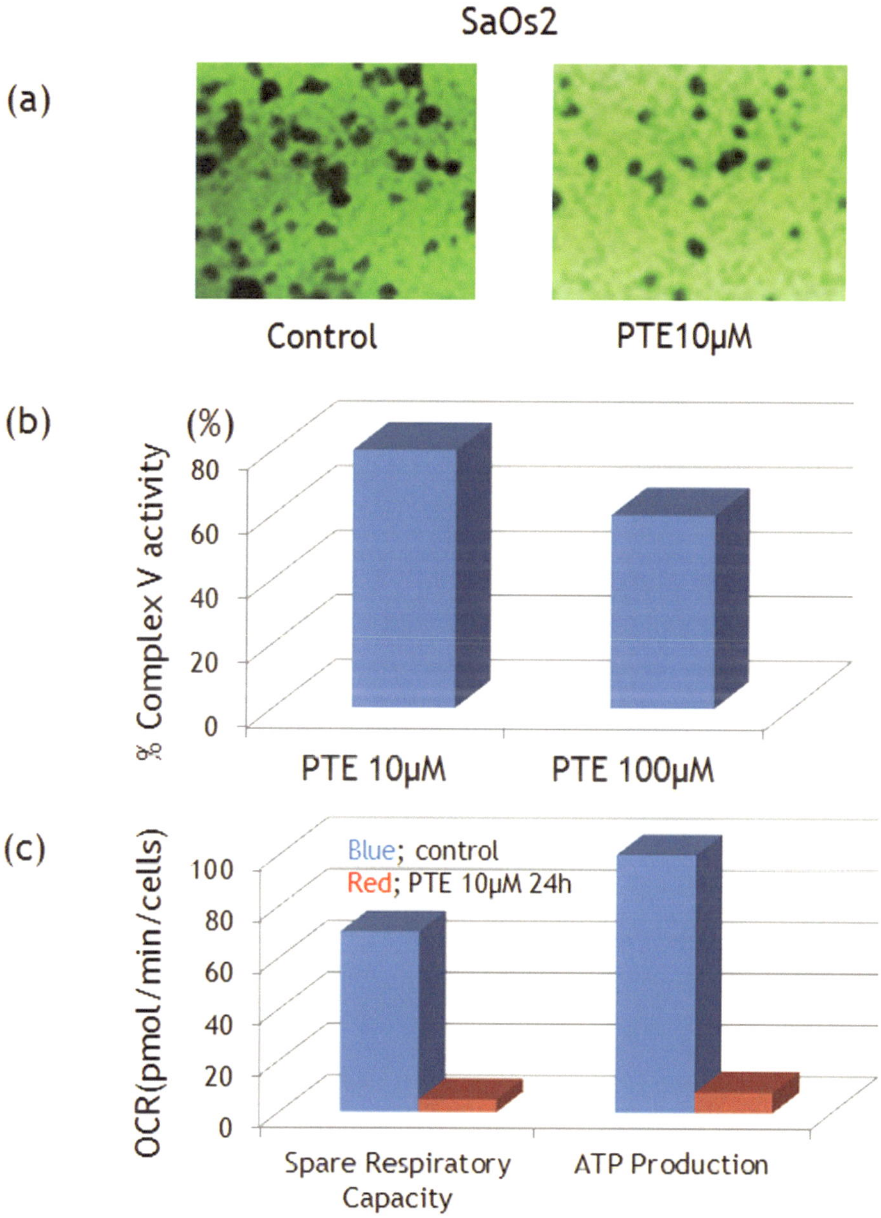

Figure 4.
(a) Pterostilbene (PTE) treatment on human osteosarcoma cells reduced the ability of sphere formation in terms of sphere number and size. (b) PTE reduced the activity of FoF1-ATP synthase, Complex V. (c) The mitochondrial OCR rates and synthetic amount of ATP were also decreased in spheroid condition (Kishi et al. unpublished data).

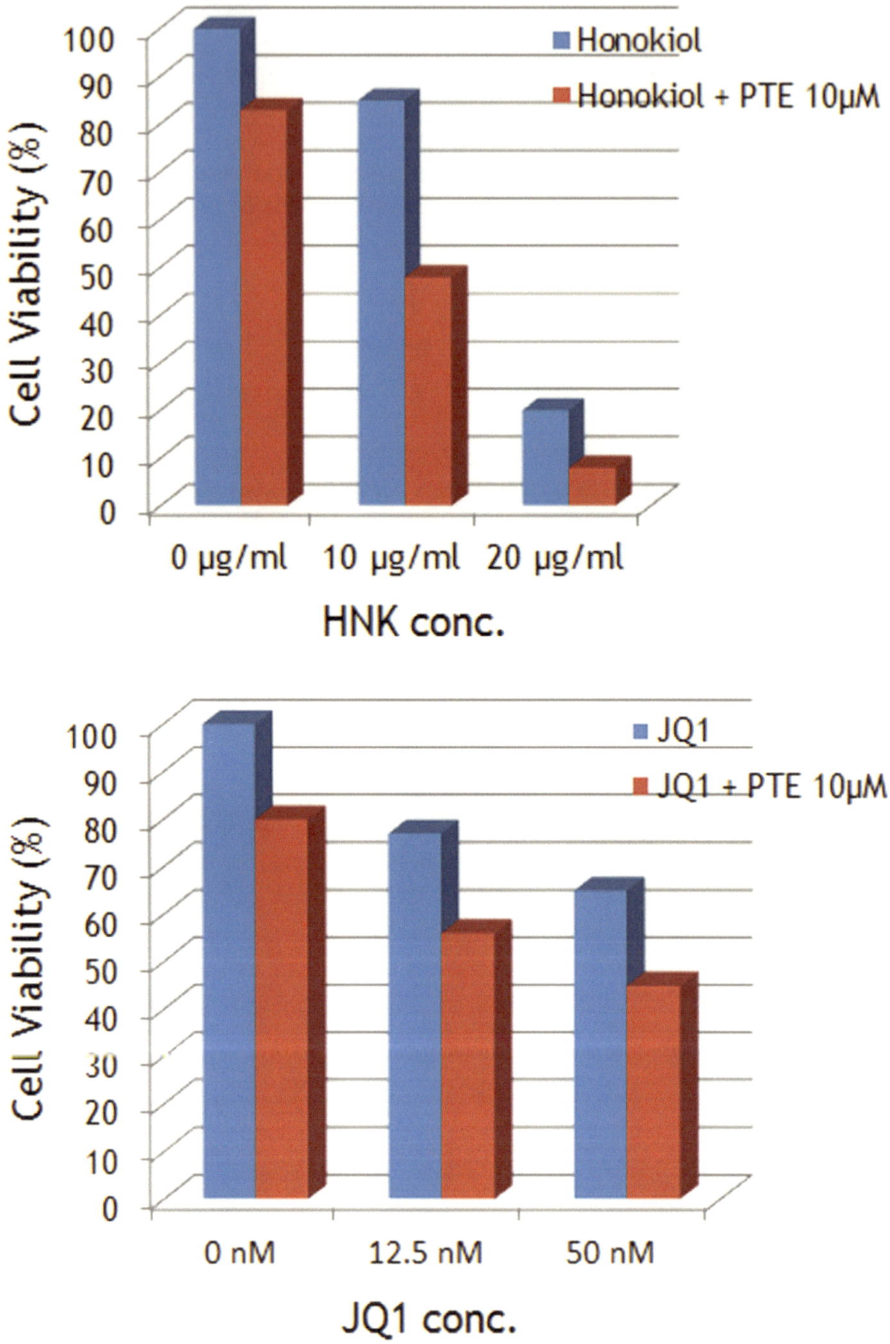

Figure 5.
Dual inhibition of OXPHOS by PTE and c-Myc inhibition by Honokiol (HNK) or JQ1 showed the synergistic effect on inhibition of osteosarcoma cell growth in a dose-dependent manner (Kishi et al. unpublished data).

The above results suggested that c-Myc inhibitor could lead to metabolic flux to OXPHOS and PTE could lead to metabolic flux to glycolysis. Thus, these exerted a great synergistic effect with "two metabolic hits" or "dual metabolic inhibition" of distinct metabolic features, OXPHOS and glycolysis, and it could be a novel therapeutic strategy against osteosarcoma, possibly targeting both stemlike cell population and general tumor cell population.

6. Conclusions

Prognosis of the patients with osteosarcoma has been improved; actually, we could say "dramatically," over the last quarter-century. However, it is also true that it has reached to plateau without any breakthroughs, and nearly 30% of patients still have to face very severe poor prognosis, especially with metastatic disease. We need to develop a novel treatment to combat such a poor prognostic situation. Targeting the distinct metabolic features of OXPHOS and glycolysis with the concept of "two metabolic hits"/"dual metabolic inhibition" strategy could bring a new insight into the field of osteosarcoma treatment, and some natural compounds such as pterostilbene and honokiol could be the possible candidates to achieve this aim.

Acknowledgements

This article is supported by a part of the Grant to KH (No. 15K10455 from the Ministry of Sports, Culture, Education, Science and Technology, Japan).

Conflict of interest

All authors have no "conflict of interest" to be declared.

Author details

Shingo Kishi[1,2], Kanya Honoki[2]*, Yasuhito Tanaka[2] and Hiroki Kuniyasu[1]

1 Department of Molecular Pathology, Nara Medical University, Kashihara, Japan

2 Department of Orthopedic Surgery, Nara Medical University, Kashihara, Japan

*Address all correspondence to: kahonoki@naramed-u.ac.jp

References

[1] Bonnet D, Dick JE. Human acute myeloid leukemia is organized as a hierarchy that originates from a primitive hematopoietic cell. Nature Medicine. 1997;**3**:730-737

[2] Al-Hajj M, Wicha MS, Benito-Hernandez A, Morrison SJ, Clarke MF. Prospective identification of tumorigenic breast cancer cells. Proceedings of the National Academy of Sciences of the United States of America. 2003;**100**:3983-3988

[3] Singh SK, Hawkins C, Clarke ID, Squire JA, Bayani J, Hide T, et al. Identification of human brain tumour initiating cells. Nature. 2004;**432**:396-401

[4] Gibbs CP, Kukekov VG, Reith JD, Tchigrinova O, Suslov ON, Scott EW, et al. Stem-like cells in bone sarcomas: Implications for tumorigenesis. Neoplasia. 2005;**7**:967-976

[5] Fujii H, Honoki K, Tsujiuchi T, Kido A, Yoshitani K, Takakura Y. Sphere-forming stem-like cell populations with drug resistance in human sarcoma cell lines. International Journal of Oncology. 2009;**34**:1381-1386

[6] Honoki K, Fujii H, Kubo A, Kido A, Mori T, Tanaka Y, et al. Possible involvement of stem-like populations with elevated ALDH1 in sarcomas for chemotherapeutic drug resistance. Oncology Reports. 2010;**24**:501-505

[7] Li C, Heidt DG, Dalerba P, Burant CF, Zhang L, Adsay V, et al. Identification of pancreatic cancer stem cells. Cancer Research. 2007;**67**:1030-1037

[8] Hermann PC, Huber SL, Herrler T, Aicher A, Ellwart JW, Guba M, et al. Distinct populations of cancer stem cells determine tumor growth and metastatic activity in human pancreatic cancer. Cell Stem Cell. 2007;**1**:313-323

[9] Lonardo E, Hermann PC, Mueller MT, Huber S, Balic A, Miranda-Lorenzo I, et al. Nodal/activin signaling drives self-renewal and tumorigenicity of pancreatic cancer stem cells and provides a target for combined drug therapy. Cell Stem Cell. 2011;**9**:433-446

[10] Vander Heiden MG, Cantley LC, Thompson CB. Understanding the Warburg effect: The metabolic requirements of cell proliferation. Science. 2009;**324**:1029-1033

[11] Dong C, Yuan T, Wu Y, Wang Y, Fan TW, Miriyala S, et al. Loss of FBP1 by snail-mediated repression provides metabolic advantages in basal-like breast cancer. Cancer Cell. 2013;**23**:316-331

[12] Li F, Wang Y, Zeller KI, Potter JJ, Wonsey DR, O'Donnell KA, et al. Myc stimulates nuclearly encoded mitochondrial genes and mitochondrial biogenesis. Molecular and Cellular Biology. 2005;**25**:6225-6234

[13] Folmes CD, Dzeja PP, Nelson TJ, Terzic A. Metabolic plasticity in stem cell homeostasis and differentiation. Cell Stem Cell. 2012;**11**:596-606

[14] Shen YA, Wang CY, Hsieh YT, Chen YJ, Wei YH. Metabolic reprogramming orchestrates cancer stem cell properties in nasopharyngeal carcinoma. Cell Cycle. 2015;**14**:86-98

[15] Ye XQ, Li Q, Wang GH, Sun FF, Huang GJ, Bian XW, et al. Mitochondrial and energy metabolism-related properties as novel indicators of lung cancer stem cells. International Journal of Cancer. 2011;**129**:820-831

[16] Janiszewska M, Suvà ML, Riggi N, Houtkooper RH, Auwerx J, Clément-Schatlo V, et al. Imp2 controls oxidative phosphorylation and is crucial for preserving glioblastoma cancer

stem cells. Genes & Development. 2012;**26**:1926-1944

[17] Sancho P, Burgos-Ramos E, Tavera A, Bou Kheir T, Jagust P, Schoenhals M, et al. MYC/PGC-1α balance determines the metabolic phenotype and plasticity of pancreatic cancer stem cells. Cell Metabolism. 2015;**22**:590-605

[18] Palorini R, Votta G, Balestrieri C, Monestiroli A, Olivieri S, Vento R, et al. Energy metabolism characterization of a novel cancer stem cell-like line 3AB-OS. Journal of Cellular Biochemistry. 2014;**115**:368-379

[19] Funes JM, Quintero M, Henderson S, Martinez D, Qureshi U, Westwood C, et al. Transformation of human mesenchymal stem cells increases their dependency on oxidative phosphorylation for energy production. Proceedings of the National Academy of Sciences of the United States of America. 2007;**104**:6223-6228

[20] Peiris-Pagès M, Martinez-Outschoorn UE, Pestell RG, Sotgia F, Lisanti MP. Cancer stem cell metabolism. Breast Cancer Research. 2016;**18**:55. DOI: 10.1186/s13058-016-0712-6

[21] Bomken S, Fišer K, Heidenreich O, Vormoor J. Understanding the cancer stem cell. British Journal of Cancer. 2010;**103**:439-445

[22] Bonuccelli G, Avnet S, Grisendi G, Salerno M, Granchi D, Dominici M, et al. Role of mesenchymal stem cells in osteosarcoma and metabolic reprogramming of tumor cells. Oncotarget. 2014;**5**:7575-7588

[23] Moore KA, Lemischka IR. Stem cells and their niches. Science. 2006;**311**:1880-1885

[24] Lamb R, Harrison H, Hulit J, Smith DL, Lisanti MP, Sotgia F. Mitochondria as new therapeutic targets for eradicating cancer stem cells: Quantitative proteomics and functional validation via MCT1/2 inhibition. Oncotarget. 2014;**5**:11029-11037

[25] Lamb R, Ozsvari B, Lisanti CL, Tanowitz HB, Howell A, Martinez-Outschoorn UE, et al. Antibiotics that target mitochondria effectively eradicate cancer stem cells, across multiple tumor types: Treating cancer like an infectious disease. Oncotarget. 2015;**6**:4569-4584

[26] Dang CV, Le A, Gao P. MYC-induced cancer cell energy metabolism and therapeutic opportunities. Clinical Cancer Research. 2009;**15**:6479-6483

[27] Kim JW, Gao P, Liu YC, Semenza GL, Dang CV. Hypoxia-inducible factor 1 and dysregulated c-Myc cooperatively induce vascular endothelial growth factor and metabolic switches hexokinase 2 and pyruvate dehydrogenase kinase 1. Molecular and Cellular Biology. 2007;**27**:7381-7393

[28] Osthus RC, Shim H, Kim S, Li Q, Reddy R, Mukherjee M, et al. Deregulation of glucose transporter 1 and glycolytic gene expression by c-Myc. The Journal of Biological Chemistry. 2000;**275**:21797-21800

[29] Le A et al. Inhibition of lactate dehydrogenase A induces oxidative stress and inhibits tumor progression. Proceedings of the National Academy of Sciences of the United States of America. 2010;**107**:2037

[30] Available from: http://www.stanford.edu/group/nusselab/cgibin/wnt/human_genetic_diseases; 2010

[31] Kim J, Woo AJ, Chu J, Snow JW, Fujiwara Y, Kim CG, et al. A myc network accounts for similarities between embryonic stem and cancer cell transcription programs. Cell. 2010;**143**:313-324

[32] Lin CY, Loven J, Rahl PB, Paranal RM, Burge CB, Bradner JE, et al.

Transcriptional amplification in tumor cells with elevated C-Myc. Cell. 2012;**151**:56-67

[33] Devi GR, Beer TM, Corless CL, Arora V, Weller DL, Iversen PL. In vivo bioavailability and pharmacokinetics of a c-MYC antisense phosphorodiamidate morpholino oligomer, AVI-4126, in solid tumors. Clinical Cancer Research. 2005;**11**:3930-3938

[34] Wang H, Mannava S, Grachtchouk V, Zhuang D, Soengas MS, Gudkov AV, et al. c-Myc depletion inhibits proliferation of human tumor cells at various stages of the cell cycle. Oncogene. 2008;**27**:1905-1915

[35] Delmore JE, Issa GC, Lemieux ME, Rahl PB, Shi J, Jacobs HM, et al. BET bromodomain inhibition as a therapeutic strategy to target c-Myc. Cell. 2011;**146**:904-917

[36] Wiegering A, Uthe FW, Jamieson T, Ruoss Y, Hüttenrauch M, Küspert M, et al. Targeting translation initiation bypasses signaling crosstalk mechanisms that maintain high myc levels in colorectal cancer. Cancer Discovery. 2015;**5**:768-781

[37] Vazquez F, Lim JH, Chim H, Bhalla K, Girnun G, Pierce K, et al. PGC1α expression defines a subset of human melanoma tumors with increased mitochondrial capacity and resistance to oxidative stress. Cancer Cell. 2013;**23**:287-301

[38] LeBleu VS, O'Connell JT, Gonzalez Herrera KN, Wikman H, Pantel K, Haigis MC, et al. PGC-1α mediates mitochondrial biogenesis and oxidative phosphorylation in cancer cells to promote metastasis. Nature Cell Biology. 2014;**16**:992-1003. 1-15

[39] Reya T, Morrison SJ, Clarke MF, Weissman IL. Stem cells, cancer, and cancer stem cells. Nature. 2001;**414**:105-111. DOI: 10.1038/35102167

[40] Chen K, Huang YH, Jl C. Understanding and targeting cancer stem cells: Therapeutic implications and challenges. Acta Pharmacologica Sinica. 2013;**34**:732-740. DOI: 10.1038/aps.2013.27

[41] Sancho P, Barneda D, Heeschen C. Hallmarks of cancer stem cell metabolism. British Journal of Cancer. 2016;**114**:1305-1312. DOI: 10.1038/bjc.2016.152

[42] Facucho-Oliveira JM, St John JC. The relationship between pluripotency and mitochondrial DNA proliferation during early embryo development and embryonic stem cell differentiation. Stem Cell Reviews. 2009;**5**:140-158. DOI: 10.1007/s12015-009-9058-0

[43] Martinez-Outschoorn UE, Peiris-Pagés M, Pestell RG, Sotgia F, Lisanti MP. Cancer metabolism: A therapeutic perspective. Nature Reviews. Clinical Oncology. 2017;**14**:113. DOI: 10.1038/nrclinonc.2017.1

[44] Vlashi E, Lagadec C, Vergnes L, Matsutani T, Masui K, Poulou M, et al. Metabolic state of glioma stem cells and nontumorigenic cells. Proceedings of the National Academy of Sciences of the United States of America. 2011;**108**:16062-16067. DOI: 10.1073/pnas.1106704108

[45] De Francesco EM, Bonuccelli G, Maggiolini M, Sotgia F, Lisanti MP. Vitamin C and doxycycline: A synthetic lethal combination therapy targeting metabolic flexibility in cancer stem cells (CSCs). Oncotarget. 2017;**8**:67269-67286. DOI: 10.18632/oncotarget.18428

[46] Lonergan T, Brenner C, Bavister B. Differentiation-related changes in mitochondrial properties as indicators of stem cell competence. Journal of Cellular Physiology. 2006;**208**:149-153

[47] Bavister BD. The mitochondrial contribution to stem cell biology.

Reproduction, Fertility, and Development. 2006;**18**:829-838

[48] Sauer H, Wartenberg M. Reactive oxygen species as signaling molecules in cardiovascular differentiation of embryonic stem cells and tumor-induced angiogenesis. Antioxidants & Redox Signaling. 2005;7:1423-1434

[49] Plotnikov EY, Marei MV, Podgornyi OV, Aleksandrova MA, Zorov DB, Sukhikh GT. Functional activity of mitochondria in cultured neural precursor cells. Bulletin of Experimental Biology and Medicine. 2006;**141**:142-146

[50] Kucia M, Ratajczak MZ. Stem cells as a two edged sword—From regeneration to tumor formation. Journal of Physiology and Pharmacology. 2006;**57**(Suppl 7):5-16

[51] Hirsch HA, Iliopoulos D, Struhl K. Metformin inhibits the inflammatory response associated with cellular transformation and cancer stem cell growth. Proceedings of the National Academy of Sciences of the United States of America. 2013;**110**:972-977. DOI: 10.1073/pnas.1221055110

[52] Fiorillo M, Lamb R, Tanowitz HB, Mutti L, Krstic-Demonacos M, Cappello AR, et al. Repurposing atovaquone: Targeting mitochondrial complex III and OXPHOS to eradicate cancer stem cells. Oncotarget. 2016;7:34084-34099. DOI: 10.18632/oncotarget.9122

[53] Alvero AB, Montagna MK, Holmberg JC, Craveiro V, Brown D, Mor G. Targeting the mitochondria activates two independent cell death pathways in ovarian cancer stem cells. Molecular Cancer Therapeutics. 2011;**10**:1385-1393. DOI: 10.1158/1535-7163.MCT-11-0023

[54] Biasutto L, Dong LF, Zoratti M, Neuzil J. Mitochondrially targeted anti-cancer agents. Mitochondrion. 2010;**10**:670-681. DOI: 10.1016/j.mito.2010.06.004

[55] Fulda S, Galluzzi L, Kroemer G. Targeting mitochondria for cancer therapy. Nature Reviews. Drug Discovery. 2010;**9**:447-464. DOI: 10.1038/nrd3137

[56] Cheong JH, Park ES, Liang J, Dennison JB, Tsavachidou D, Nguyen-Charles C, et al. Dual inhibition of tumor energy pathway by 2-deoxyglucose and metformin is effective against a broad spectrum of preclinical cancer models. Molecular Cancer Therapeutics. 2011;**10**:2350-2362. DOI: 10.1158/1535-7163.MCT-11-0497

[57] Issaq SH, Teicher BA, Monks A. Bioenergetic properties of human sarcoma cells help define sensitivity to metabolic inhibitors. Cell Cycle. 2014;**13**:1152-1161. DOI: 10.4161/cc.28010

[58] Kang JH, Lee SH, Lee JS, Nam B, Seong TW, Son J, et al. Aldehyde dehydrogenase inhibition combined with phenformin treatment reversed NSCLC through ATP depletion. Oncotarget. 2016;7:49397-49410

[59] Loureiro R, Mesquita KA, Oliveira PJ, Vega-Naredo I. Mitochondria in cancer stem cells: A target for therapy. Recent Patents on Endocrine, Metabolic & Immune Drug Discovery. 2013;7:102-114

[60] Pathania D, Millard M, Neamati N. Opportunities in discovery and delivery of anticancer drugs targeting mitochondria and cancer cell metabolism. Advanced Drug Delivery Reviews. 2009;**61**:1250-1275. DOI: 10.1016/j.addr.2009.05.010

[61] Ghadially FN, Mehta PN. Ultrastructure of osteogenic sarcoma. Cancer. 1970;**25**:1457-1467

[62] Singh I, Tsang KY, Ludwig GD. Alterations in the mitochondria of human osteosarcoma cells with

glucocorticoids. Cancer Research. 1974;**34**:2946-2952

[63] Giang AH, Raymond T, Brookes P, de Mesy Bentley K, Schwarz E, O'Keefe R, et al. Mitochondrial dysfunction and permeability transition in osteosarcoma cells showing the Warburg effect. The Journal of Biological Chemistry. 2013;**288**:33303-33311. DOI: 10.1074/jbc.M113.507129

[64] Sánchez-Cenizo L, Formentini L, Aldea M, Ortega AD, García-Huerta P, Sánchez-Aragó M, et al. Up-regulation of the ATPase inhibitory factor 1 (IF1) of the mitochondrial H^+-ATP synthase in human tumors mediates the metabolic shift of cancer cells to a Warburg phenotype. The Journal of Biological Chemistry. 2010;**285**:25308-25313. DOI: 10.1074/jbc.M110.146480

[65] Barbato S, Sgarbi G, Gorini G, Baracca A, Solaini G. The inhibitor protein (IF1) of the F1F0-ATPase modulates human osteosarcoma cell bioenergetics. The Journal of Biological Chemistry. 2015;**290**:6338-6348. DOI: 10.1074/jbc.M114.631788

[66] Dandawate P, Padhye S, Ahmad A, Sarkar FH. Novel strategies targeting cancer stem cells through phytochemicals and their analogs. Drug Delivery and Translational Research. 2013;**3**:165-182. DOI: 10.1007/s13346-012-0079-x

[67] Singh AK, Sharma N, Ghosh M, Park YH, Jeong DK. Emerging importance of dietary phytochemicals in fight against cancer: Role in targeting cancer stem cells. Critical Reviews in Food Science and Nutrition. 2017;**57**:3449-3463. DOI: 10.1080/10408398.2015.1129310

[68] Mak KK, Wu AT, Lee WH, Chang TC, Chiou JF, Wang LS, et al. Pterostilbene, a bioactive component of blueberries, suppresses the generation of breast cancer stem cells within tumor microenvironment and metastasis via modulating NF-κB/microRNA 448 circuit. Molecular Nutrition & Food Research. 2013;**57**:1123-1134. DOI: 10.1002/mnfr.201200549

[69] Huynh TT, Lin CM, Lee WH, Wu AT, Lin YK, Lin YF, et al. Pterostilbene suppressed irradiation-resistant glioma stem cells by modulating GRP78/miR-205 axis. Journal of Nutritional Biochemistry. 2015;**26**:466-475. DOI: 10.1016/j.jnutbio.2014.11.015

[70] Lee CM, Su YH, Huynh TT, Lee WH, Chiou JF, Lin YK, et al. Blueberry isolate, pterostilbene, functions as a potential anticancer stem cell agent in suppressing irradiation-mediated enrichment of hepatoma stem cells. Evidence-Based Complementary and Alternative Medicine. 2013;**2013**:258425. DOI: 10.1155/2013/258425

[71] Huang WC, Chan ML, Chen MJ, Tsai TH, Chen YJ. Modulation of macrophage polarization and lung cancer cell stemness by MUC1 and development of a related small-molecule inhibitor pterostilbene. Oncotarget. 2016;**7**:39363-39375. DOI: 10.18632/oncotarget.8101

[72] Li Z, Dong H, Li M, Wu Y, Liu Y, Zhao Y, et al. Honokiol induces autophagy and apoptosis of osteosarcoma through PI3K/Akt/mTOR signaling pathway. Molecular Medicine Reports. 2018;**17**:2719-2723. DOI: 10.3892/mmr.2017.8123

[73] Yao CJ, Lai GM, Yeh CT, Lai MT, Shih PH, Chao WJ, et al. Honokiol eliminates human oral cancer stem-like cells accompanied with suppression of Wnt/β-catenin signaling and apoptosis induction. Evidence-based Complementary and Alternative Medicine. 2013;**2013**:146136. DOI: 10.1155/2013/146136

[74] Hahm ER, Singh KB, Singh SV. c-Myc is a novel target of cell cycle arrest by honokiol in prostate cancer cells. Cell Cycle. 2016;**15**(17):2309-2320. DOI: 10.1080/15384101.2016.1201253

Chapter 5

Treatment of Children with Osteosarcoma

Maxim Yu. Rykov and Elmira R. Sengapova

Abstract

Osteosarcoma accounts for 3% of all malignant tumors, 35–50% of all malignant bone tumors in pediatric patients. The chapter contains statistical data describing the incidence of the child population of osteosarcomas, classification of osteosarcomas, staging principles, a description of the main localizations, as well as a detailed description of the existing treatment protocols for children with osteosarcomas, including personalized therapy. The literature data are described in detail—the results of treatment of children with osteosarcoma with various courses of chemotherapy, as well as new approaches in treatment, including personalized therapy. But the results of treatment of children with primary metastatic osteosarcoma, relapse, and refractory course of the disease remain unsatisfactory.

Keywords: pediatric oncology, osteosarcoma, chemotherapy, personalized therapy, combination treatment

1. Introduction

Osteosarcoma is a primary malignant bone tumor that develops from primitive mesenchymal stem cells capable of differentiating into bone, cartilage, or fibrous tissue [1].

Osteosarcoma accounts for 3% of all malignant tumors, 35–50% of all malignant bone tumors in pediatric patients. The frequency of occurrence is 4 cases per 1 million children and adolescents per year. About 60% of cases of osteosarcoma detection are recorded at the age of 10–20 years (mainly in the prepubertal and pubertal periods). The gender ratio (boys/girls) is 1.3–1.6:1 [2].In 50% of cases, the tumor is located in the projection of the knee joint (distal femur, proximal tibial bone). The third place in terms of frequency of occurrence is the lesion of the proximal metadiaphysis of the humerus. The defeat of the axial skeleton (pelvis, spinal column) is detected in 12% of cases [3–5].

In the treatment of children with osteosarcoma, chemotherapy is the main method. Nonadjuvant and adjuvant chemotherapy courses are important. In the middle of the twentieth century, when the main treatment was surgical, the frequency of relapse and metastasis was extremely high. Increased patient survival is due precisely to the intensification of chemotherapeutic treatment, which has reduced the frequency of relapses and metastasis.

2. Classification and staging

2.1 WHO classification of soft tissue and bone tumors of 2013 (fourth revision)

A localized (locally advanced) variant of osteosarcoma, which occurs in 80% of cases and a disseminated (primary metastatic) variant, which occurs in 20% of cases, are distinguished [3, 6].

2.2 Histological classification

- low grade, central osteosarcoma
- classic (conventional) version of osteosarcoma:
    - chondroblastic osteosarcoma
    - fibroblastic osteosarcoma
    - osteoblastic osteosarcoma
    - osteosarcoma, unspecified accuracy
- telangiectatic osteosarcoma
- small cell osteosarcoma
- high degree of malignancy, superficial osteosarcoma.

2.3 TNM classification 2018:

2.3.1 TNM classification 2018 for the extremities

T—primary tumor
Tx—the primary tumor cannot be determined [7].
T0—no signs of primary tumor.
T1—the largest tumor size ≤8 cm.
T2—the largest tumor size>8 cm.
T3—several unrelated tumors in the primary zone of bone damage.
N—regional lymph nodes:
Nx—the presence of metastatic lesions in the regional lymph nodes cannot be determined.
N0—no regional metastases in the lymph nodes.
N1—regional lymph node metastases.
M—distant metastases:
Mx—the presence of distant metastases could not be determined or the study was not conducted.
M0—distant metastases are absent.
M1—there are distant metastases.
M1a—in the lungs.
M1b—another localization.
G—degree of differentiation:
Gx—the degree of differentiation could not be determined or the study was not conducted.

G1—well differentiated.
G2—moderately differentiated.
G3—poorly differentiated.
G4—undifferentiated.
G1–2—low degree of malignancy.
G3–4—a high degree of malignancy.

2.3.2 TNM classification 2018 for the spine

TX	Primary tumor cannot be assessed
T0	No evidence of primary tumor
T1	Tumor confined to one vertebral segment or two adjacent vertebral segments
T2	Tumor confined to three adjacent vertebral segments
T3	Tumor confined to four or more adjacent vertebral segments, or any nonadjacent vertebral segments
T4	Extension into the spinal canal or great vessels
T4a	Extension into the spinal canal
T4b	Evidence of gross vascular invasion or tumor thrombus in the great vessels
NX	Regional lymph nodes cannot be assessed. Because of the rarity of lymph node involvement in bone sarcomas, the designation NX may not be appropriate, and cases should be considered N0 unless clinical node involvement clearly is evident
N0	No regional lymph node metastasis
N1	Regional lymph node metastasis
cM0	No distant metastasis
cM1	Distant metastasis
cM1a	Lung
cM1b	Bone or other distant sites
pM1	Distant metastasis, microscopically confirmed
cM1a	Lung, microscopically confirmed
cM1b	Bone or other distant sites. Microscopically confirmed

2.3.3 TNM classification 2018 for the pelvis

TX	Primary tumor cannot be assessed
T0	No evidence of primary tumor
T1	Tumor confined to one pelvic segment with no extraosseous extension
T1a	Tumor ≤8 cm in greatest dimension
T1b	Tumor >8 cm in greatest dimension
T2	Tumor confined to one pelvic segment with extraosseous extension or two segments without extraosseous extension
T2a	Tumor ≤8 cm in greatest dimension
T2b	Tumor >8 cm in greatest dimension
T3	Tumor spanning two pelvic segments with extraosseous extension
T3a	Tumor ≤8 cm in greatest dimension
T3b	Tumor >8 cm in greatest dimension

T4	Tumor spanning three pelvic segments or crossing the sacroiliac joint
T4a	Tumor involves sacroiliac joint and extends medial to the sacral neuroforamen
T4b	Tumor encasement of external iliac vessels or presence of gross tumor thrombus in major pelvic vessels
NX	Regional lymph nodes cannot be assessed. Because of the rarity of lymph node involvement in bone sarcomas, the designation NX may not be appropriate, and cases should be considered N0 unless clinical node involvement clearly is evident
N0	No regional lymph node metastasis
N1	Regional lymph node metastasis
cM0	No distant metastasis
cM1	Distant metastasis
cM1a	Lung
cM1b	Bone or other distant sites
pM1	Distant metastasis, microscopically confirmed
cM1a	Lung, microscopically confirmed
cM1b	Bone or other distant sites. Microscopically confirmed

Stage	TNM	Degree of malignancy
IA	T1 N0 M0	Low
IB	T2 N0 M0	Low
IIA	T1 N0 M0	High
IIB	T2 N0 M0	High
III	T3 N0 M0	Any
IVA	Any T N0 M1a	Any
IVB	Any T N1 Any M Any T Any N M1b	Any Any

Table 1.
Staging by TNM.

Staging according to the TNM classification is presented in **Table 1**.

3. Treatment

The methods of treatment of osteosarcoma over the past 30 years have not changed. There are five main drugs (cisplatin, adriamycin, methotrexate, ifosfamide, and etoposide) that have been used in various combinations and doses [8–13].

The rates of treatment outcome in the world remain at about the same level. In patients with a localized variant of osteosarcoma, 5-year overall survival (OS) does not exceed 75% and 5-year event-free survival (EFS)—62% (**Table 2**).

In patients with primary metastatic osteosarcoma, the results are much worse, despite attempts to use high doses of drugs, including high-dose polychemotherapy with transplantation of autologous hematopoietic stem cells. At the same time, the 5-year OS does not exceed 35% on average and the 5-year EFS–25% (**Table 2**).

Therapy program	5-year overall survival, %	5-year event-free survival, %
IOR/OS2 the Istituto Ortopedico Rizzoli [14]	75	63
ISG/OS1 (Italian Sarcoma Group) [15]	74	64
ISG/SSG1 (Italian and Scandinavian Sarcoma Group) [16]	77	64
COSS 88/96 (Cooperative Osteosarcoma Study Group) [17]	79	
SSG XIV (Scandinavian Sarcoma Group) [18]		65
NECO93J/95J (Neoadjuvant Chemotherapy for Osteosarcoma) [19]	78	65
BOTG III/IV (Brazilian Osteosarcoma Treatment Group) [20]	61	45
POG8651 (Pediatric Oncology Group) [21]	78	65
SFOP94 (Société Française d'Oncologie Pédiatrique) [22]	76	62
St.Jude CRH OS91 (Children Research Hospital) [23]	74	65
St.Jude CRH OS99 (Children Research Hospital) [24]	79	67
INT0133-COG (+MTP/-MTP) Children's Oncology Group [25]	78/70	67/61
MSKC NY (+PAM) Memorial Sloan-Kettering Cancer Center, NY [26]	94	72
COG INT0133, CCG7943, AOST0121 [27]	47	22
ISG/SSG II (Italian and Scandinavian Sarcoma Group) [28]	55	46
EURAMOS1 [29, 30]	75	59

Table 2.
The results of the treatment of pediatric patients with localized osteosarcoma.

3.1 Traditional treatment

The most significant interest in the treatment of children with a localized version of osteosarcoma are the studies of the Italian and Scandinavian groups (Italian and Scandinavian sarcoma group–ISG/SSGI, SSG XIV), the French Pediatric Oncological Group (Societe Francaise d'Oncologie Pediatrique–SFOP OS94), and EURAMOS1.

Ferrari et al. showed the data of the joint study of the Italian and Scandinavian groups (ISG/SSG I), which was conducted from 1997 to 2000. The study included 182 patients.

A special feature of neoadjuvant chemotherapy was the use of two courses of monotherapy with high dose ifosfamide (in a course dose of 15 g/m^2) and two courses of MAR (methotrexate (M) 12 g/m^2, adriamycin (A) 75 mg/m^2, and cisplatin (P) 120 mg/m^2) in alternating mode. Adjuvant chemotherapy started at week 14. In this case, the course dose of adriamycin was increased to 90 mg/m^2, the dose of cisplatin to 150 mg/m^2, and a high-dose ifosfamide was administered in PIM chemotherapy courses (cisplatin, ifosfamide, and methotrexate) and PAI (cisplatin, adriamycin, and ifosfamide).

After removal of the primary tumor focus, a good histological response (therapeutic pathomorphism of grade 3–4) was achieved in 63% of patients, a poor histological response (treatment pathomorphism of grade 1–2) in 37%. At the same time, the 5-year OV and EFS accounted for 77 and 64%. Consequently, the use of high-dose ifosfamide in an alternating mode with the MAP scheme led to an increase in the frequency of achieving a good histological response, but did not affect the rates of OS and EFS [15, 16, 31].

Smeland et al. presented the data of the study of the Scandinavian Group (SSG XIV), which was conducted from 2001 to 2005. The study included 63 patients.

Neoadjuvant chemotherapy consisted of two courses of IDA. High-dose ifosfamide (in the course dose of 10 g/m^2) was used in monotherapy in patients with a poor histological response to treatment, only after five courses of MAP.

After removal of the primary tumor lesion, a good histological response was achieved in 45% of patients and a poor histological response in 55%. At the same time, the 5-year OV and BSV accounted for 76–65% and the 5-year EFS in the group with a good histological response for 89%, with a poor histological response 48%. Consequently, the use of ifosfamide after MAP courses in the adjuvant mode did not lead to an increase in OS and EFS, and the frequency of achieving a good histological response was lower than in studies in which the MAP scheme was used in alternating mode with ifosfamide [18].

Le Deley et al. presented the results of the randomized SFOP OS94 study, which was conducted from 1994 to 2001. The study included 239 patients (120 in group A and 119 in group B).

Neoadjuvant therapy included seven courses of high-dose methotrexate and two courses of monotherapy with adriamycin (in a course dose of 70 mg/m^2) in group A or seven courses of high-dose methotrexate and two courses of IE (ifosfamide (I) 12 g/m^2 and etoposide (E) 300 mg/m^2) in group B. In the adjuvant mode, chemotherapy was replaced with IE courses in group A, and AP in group B for patients with a poor histological response detected after removal of the primary focus. The operative stage of treatment was carried out at 12 and 14 weeks in groups A and B, respectively.

A good histological response was achieved in group A in 43% of patients, in group B in 64%, poor histological response in group A in 57%, and in group B in 36% ($p = 0.009$). The 5-year OS in group A was 75%, in group B—76%, the 5-year EFS in group A—58%, and in group B—66%. A 3-year EFS in group A in patients showed a good histological response for 82%, with a poor histological response for 49%, in group B—77 and 60%, respectively.

Consequently, the use of methotrexate, ifosfamide and etoposide in neoadjuvant chemotherapy led to a statistically significant increase in the frequency of achieving a good histological response, but not to an increase in OS and EFS [22].

Of particular interest in the treatment of children with primary metastatic osteosarcoma are the Pediatric Oncology Group (POG) IE and ISG/SSG II studies.

Goorin et al. presented the results of a phase II/III nonrandomized clinical trial of high-dose ifosfamide and etoposide in patients with primary metastatic osteosarcoma. The study included 43 patients.

Neoadjuvant chemotherapy was represented by two courses of IE (ifosfamide (I) 17.5 g/m^2 and etoposide (E) 500 mg/m^2). Removal of the primary tumor lesion was performed after two courses of IE at 7–8 weeks of therapy. The timing of the removal of metastatic foci was chosen individually during adjuvant chemotherapy, which included four courses of MAP chemotherapy and three courses of iE (with a course dose of ifosfamide (i) 12 g/m^2) in an alternating mode.

A good histological response was achieved in 65% of patients and poor in 35%. However, the 2-year OS and EFS were 55 and 45%, respectively. Consequently, the use of high-dose ifosfamide in combination with etoposide therapy led to an increase in the frequency of achieving a good histological response, but not indicators of OS and EFS [32].

Boye et al. showed the results of the nonrandomized study ISG/SSG II, which was conducted from 1996 to 2004. The study included 57 patients with primary metastatic osteosarcoma.

Neoadjuvant chemotherapy included two courses of MAPI. Surgical removal of the primary tumor lesion was performed at week 14.

In the adjuvant mode, two courses of ACyVP (adriamycin (A) 90 mg/m^2, cyclophosphamide (Cy) 4 g/m^2, and vepesid (VP) 600 mg/m^2) and two courses of high-dose chemotherapy VPCarbo (vepesid (VP) 600 mg/m^2 and carboplatin (Carbo) 1.5 g/m^2) with the support of autologous hematopoietic stem cells. Surgical removal of the primary tumor lesion was performed at week 14.

A good histological response was achieved in 29% of patients and poor in 71%. The 5-year OM and BSV were 31 and 27%, respectively [28].

Marina et al. presented the results of the EURAMOS1 study in patients with a poor histological response after neoadjuvant MAP chemotherapy. Within the protocol, patients are randomly assigned to the MAP treatment lines (methotrexate (M) 12 g/m^2, adriamycin (A) 75 mg/m^2, and cisplatin (P) 120 mg/m^2) and MAPIE (ifosfamide (I) 14 g/m^2 and etoposide 500 mg/m^2). In the age group up to 30 years, the MAPIE line of therapy was carried out in 310 patients, the MAPIE line in 308 patients, in the age group up to 20 years—259 (84%) and 271 (88%) patients. Groups of patients are statistically significantly comparable by sex, age, localization of the primary tumor lesion, the presence of metastatic lesions, and the histological variant of the tumor.

In the group of 541 patients with a localized version of osteosarcoma, 247 events were identified, 118 in patients who received the MAP therapy line and 129 in patients who received the MAPIE therapy line. At the same time, the 3-year EFS was 60 and 57%. In the group of patients with primary metastatic osteosarcoma, 3-year EFS was 24 and 18%, for MAP and MAPIE, respectively. Therefore, this study showed that the use of alternating chemotherapy courses for MAP, IE, and Ai in an adjuvant regimen did not lead to an increase in EFS indices [33].

3.2 Experimental treatment

Treatment outcomes for children with primary metastatic osteosarcoma remain extremely low and the optimal therapeutic strategy is unknown.

New programs are being developed around the world taking into account the molecular biological features of tumor cells that determine sensitivity to chemotherapy (ERCC1 to cisplatin, TOPO2α to anthracyclines and etoposide, MGMT to epigenetic therapy and cisplatin, RFC1 to methotrexate) [34–39] and invasive and metastatic potential of a tumor (stem cell markers—CD133, OCT4; transcription factors—p-STAT3, C-MYC; cytokine-associated signaling pathways—ErbB2, VEGFR1, VEGFR2, PDGFRα, and PDGFRβ) [40–43].

Cui et al. presented the results of a study to determine the expression of MGMT protein (methylguanine–DNA–methyltransferase) and MGMT gene methylation in patients with osteosarcoma in the age group up to 40 years (mean age 17 years) who were treated with cisplatin in single mode, in a course dose of 120 mg/m^2 Determination of MGMT protein expression in immunohistochemical (IHC) study was performed in biopsy tumor material in 76 patients and MGMT gene methylation in 51 patients. The result of IHC was considered positive with a high level of expression—more than 30% (3+), with an average level of expression—20–30% (2+), and with a low level of expression—10–20% (1+). MGMT protein expression was detected in 52 (68%) patients, low expression level in 27 (35%), medium level in 18 (24%), and high level in 7 (9%).

A statistically significant relationship was established between the presence of MGMT protein expression and an increase in the frequency of a poor histological response ($p = 0.004$). The expression level above 20% was detected in 22 out of 43 (51%) patients in the group of patients with 1–2°of therapeutic pathomorphosis and only in 3 out of 33 (9%) patients in the group with 3–4° of therapeutic pathomorphosis.

Methylation of the promoter portion of the MGMT gene was observed in 12 of 51 (23.5%) patients and the lack of expression of MGMT protein in 14 of 51 (27.5%) patients. A statistically significant relationship between the absence of methylation and the presence of MGMT protein expression ($p < 0.001$) was established. In the group of patients with 1–2 degrees of therapeutic pathomorphosis, the absence of MGMT gene methylation was detected in 36 of 38 (94.7%) patients and with 3–4 degrees of therapeutic pathomorphosis in 3 of 13 (23%) patients ($p < 0.001$).

Consequently, the data obtained indicate the formation of tumor resistance to treatment with an alkylating agent—cisplatin in patients whose biopsy material revealed the absence of methylation of the promoter portion of the MGMT gene and the presence of expression of the MGMT protein [34, 35].

Pitano-Garcia et al. (Spain sarcoma group) conducted a study to determine the expression of RFC1 micro-RNA (reduced folate carrier 1, a transmembrane protein that provides folate and methotrexate transport to the cell) by real-time polymerase chain reaction (PCR) in a tumor substrate in children with osteosarcoma.

In 34 samples, biopsy tumor material in 14 children and metastatic foci tumor material in 20 children were analyzed. In 13 of 14 (92.9%) biopsy specimens and in 11 of 20 (68.8%) metastatic specimens, a low level of RFC1 expression was detected.

A poor histological response after neoadjuvant chemotherapy (three courses of intravenous administration of doxorubicin at a dose of 75 mg/m^2, three courses of intraarterial administration of cisplatin at a dose of 105 mg/m^2, four courses of intravenous administration of methotrexate at a dose of 14 g/m^2) in 45% of cases. The biopsy tumor substrate in this group of patients was characterized by a low level of expression of RFC1 micro-RNA in 90% of cases compared to 60% in patients with a good histological response ($p = 0.053$). The average level of expression was statistically significantly lower in the biopsy material than in the metastatic tumor foci ($p = 0.024$) [38, 44].

Therefore, in this study, there was a tendency to an increase in the frequency of detection of low expression levels of RFC1 micro-RNA in patients with a poor histological response.

Hattinger et al. (Italian sarcoma group) presented the results of the study, the purpose of which was to determine the prognostic significance of ERCC1 protein expression (excision repair crosscomplementation group 1) in biopsy tumor material in patients with localized osteosarcoma, who underwent programmed treatment of ISG/OS-oss and ISG/SSG1. A tumor sample was considered positive in the presence of a score of 2–3: score 1 (1–10% of positive nuclei), score 2 (11–50% of positive nuclei), and score 3 (more than 50% of positive nuclei).

ERCC1-positive tumor (score 2–3) was detected in 30 patients (30%). During the ISG/OS-oss program in groups of patients with ERCC1-negative/score 1 and ERCC1-positive (score 2–3), the 5-year-old OS and BSV tumor variants were 91, 38, and 57, 25% ($p = 0.001$; $p = 0.042$), with the ISG/SSG1 program–82, 64, and 69, 36% ($p = 0.022$; $p = 0.028$), and with both therapy programs–82, 50 and 62, 34% ($p < 0.001$; $p = 0.006$). Consequently, a statistically significant relationship has been established between the ERCC1-positive variant of the tumor and lower rates of 5-year OS and BSV [36].

Nguyen et al. (SFOP) presented the results of a study to determine the prognostic significance of TOP2A protein expression (topoisomerase DNA 2 alfa) and the presence of rearrangement of the TOP2A gene in biopsy tumor material in 105 children with osteosarcoma treated with the SFOP protocol OS94. Patients with a primary metastatic osteosarcoma variant accounted for 17%. After neoadjuvant chemotherapy, a good histological response was detected in 56 patients (53%) and a poor histological response in 49 (47%). Real-time PCR amplification of the

TOP2A gene and the TOP2A gene deletion were detected in 21 (21.2%) and 25 (25.3%) patients. In 53 children (53.5%), rearrangements of the TOP2A gene were not detected. A statistically significant relationship was established between the presence of the TOP2A gene rearrangement (amplification and deletion) and the presence of a good histological response after neoadjuvant polychemotherapy ($p = 0.004$). There was also a tendency to achieve lower rates of 5-year OM and BSV in patients whose tumor cells had amplified the TOP2A gene ($p = 0.09$ and 0.06). The expression of the TOR2A protein was determined in 17 patients by immunohistochemistry. Medium (2+) and high (3+) levels of expression were detected in all patients; expression was above 30% in 12 of 17 children (70.5%). There is no statistically significant relationship between the expression of the TOR2A protein above 30% and the presence of amplification or deletion of the TOP2A gene ($p > 0.05$) due to an insufficient number of observations [37].

Xiao et al. presented the results of a study of a personalized approach to the prescription of chemotherapy depending on the presence or absence of markers of drug resistance in 28 patients with localized osteosarcoma. The average age in the patient group was 20.1 g. To determine the sensitivity to chemotherapy, the following markers were used: for doxorubicin–expression of TOP2A micro-RNA, mutation of the ABCB1 gene, and mutation of the GSTP1 gene; for cisplatin–expression of microcryptal ERCC1, BRCA1, and mutation of genes XRCC1-exon6 and XRCC1-exon10, and for ifosfamide–mutation of CYP2C9 * 3.

At the same time, a high level of sensitivity to ifosfamide was detected in all patients (100%), to cisplatin in 11 out of 28 (39.2%), to doxorubicin in 6 out of 28 (21.4%); medium and high levels of sensitivity to cisplatin in 17 of 28 (60.7%), to doxorubicin in 20 of 28 (71.4%). Chemotherapy, taking into account the sensitivity of the tumor to drugs, was performed in 8 of 28 patients (28.5%). In this group, only one relapse of the disease was detected, while in the rest of the 20 patients, four relapses of the disease were detected: in one case, progression during neoadjuvant chemotherapy and in another case, fatal outcome from toxicity of therapy. The average duration of observation for groups was not indicated, and no statistically significant difference was obtained due to the insufficient number of observations [39].

In addition, the study of markers of stem tumor cells CD133 (Prominin 1) and Octamer-binding transcription factor 4 (OCT4), as well as the transcription factors signal transducer and activator of transcription 3 (STAT3), and myelocytomatosis viral oncogene homolog (C-MYC), which determines the invasive and metastatic potential of a tumor [45–47].

So in the work of He et al., there was a significant correlation between the expression of CD133 in tumor cells and a higher frequency of metastatic lesions, a lower median of overall survival. A CD133-positive variant was detected in 46 of 70 (65.7%) patients, in 6 out of 16 (37.5%) in the group with a localized osteosarcoma variant, and in 40 out of 54 (74%) in the group with the primary metastatic osteosarcoma ($p = 0.002$). The median overall survival rate was statistically significantly lower in the group with CD133-positive tumor ($p = 0.000$). When conducting the study "Transwell invasion," a significantly higher invasive potential of the CD133-positive variant of the tumor was established ($p < 0.05$). Real-time PCR established a higher level of expression of micro-RNA OCT4 in a CD133-positive variant of the tumor ($p < 0.05$) [41].

Li et al. in an experimental model on cell lines showed that about 80% of cells in a CD133-positive variant of the tumor are in the G0/G1 phases of the cell cycle ($p < 0.01$). Also, real-time PCR revealed a significantly higher level of expression of the multidrug-resistant gene (MDR1) in the CD133-positive variant of the tumor ($p < 0.05$) [48].

In the studies presented, He and Li et al., the mechanisms of drug resistance, invasion, and metastasis in case of CD133-positive variant of the tumor were established.

In the works of Tu et al., the significance of activation of the IL6R/STAT3/p-STAT3tyr705 mesenchymal stem cell signaling pathway to increase the metastatic potential of tumor cells was exemplified by the example of cell lines (Saos 2 and U2-OS). The relationship between the increased expression of p-STAT3tyr705 and increased expression of the drug resistance markers multidrug resistance protein (MRP) and MDR1 has been established. An increase in sensitivity to doxorubicin, but not to cisplatin, was also noted with inhibition of this signaling pathway [43, 49].

Han et al. using cell lines (MG63 and SAOS2) as an example showed that an increase in C-MYC expression leads to activation of the MEK–ERK signaling pathway and an increase in the expression of MMP2 and MMP9, which enhance the invasive and metastatic potential of a tumor [50].

Wu et al. investigated the prognostic significance of C-MYC expression in biopsy tumor material in 56 children with osteosarcoma who were treated with methotrexate, cisplatin, and adriamycin. Expression of the C-MYC protein was detected in 48 of 56 (85.7%) patients. A statistically significant relationship was established between the presence of C-MYC expression and a decrease in the apoptotic index ($p < 0.05$). In addition, in the group of patients with C-MYC-positive variant of the tumor and the intensity of expression, at 2+ and 3+, a significantly lower 3-year-old OM was established ($p < 0.05$) [51].

Consequently, in the works of Tu, Han, and Wu et al., the significance of transcription factors in the development of drug resistance, invasion, and metastasis of the tumor has been established.

3.3 Theoretical treatment

Innovative therapeutic approaches are used mainly in patients with metastatic osteosarcoma, relapse, and refractory course of the disease. Currently, the following key areas are distinguished: (1) the use of monoclonal antibody preparations, (2) tumor-modifying therapy using nitrogen-containing bisphosphonates, (3) the use of chemotherapeutic drugs that affect various cellular signaling pathways (multikinase inhibitors and mTOR inhibitors), and (4) the use of drugs that promote the activation of tumor-associated macrophages.

Rossi et al. presented the results of a study aimed at determining the expression of vascular endothelial growth factor (VEGF) in a biopsy tumor substrate and in tumor material after neoadvanting chemotherapy (two courses of MAP) in 16 patients with localized osteosarcoma, who received programmed treatment using the SSG XIV protocol. Four levels of expression were evaluated: negative and low–at an expression level <25%, medium—at 25–50% (1+), high—at 50–75% (2+), and very high—at>75% (3+). Medium and high levels of VEGF expression in biopsy tumor material were detected in 11 (6 in medium and 5 in high) out of 16 patients (68.7%). After neoadjuvant chemotherapy and the removal of the primary tumor site, VEGF expression was established in all samples, and there was an increase in expression in samples that were positive in the initial study.

High and very high levels of expression, increased expression after neoadjuvant chemotherapy was statistically significantly correlated with the localization of the primary tumor lesion in the femur ($p = 0.02$), with the appearance of local recurrence ($p = 0.04$) and/or early metastatic lesions in the lungs ($p = 0.04$), with a fatal outcome from the refractory course of the disease ($p = 0.04$).

Therefore, the presence of VEGF expression in the biopsy material and an increase in the expression of VEGF after neoadjuvant chemotherapy are factors for poor prognosis of the disease [42]. But this study requires the continuation of the fact that it includes a small number of patients.

In addition, Ohba et al. showed in an in vivo experiment using human osteosarcoma cell lines (TE85 and 143B) the mechanism of autocrine stimulation of tumor transformation and proliferation using the example of the VEGF/VEGFR signaling pathway. In this study, the expression of VEGF-A and VEGFR micro-RNA was evaluated [52].

Currently, little experience has been gained with the use of the drug bevacizumab in children with osteosarcoma.

Bevacizumab (Avastin) is a partially humanized monoclonal antibody to VEGF-A, IgG1, which realizes its activity through a second type of immunopathological reaction (antibody-mediated complement-dependent cytotoxicity and antibody-mediated cell-dependent cytotoxicity) [53].

Turner et al. (St. Jude Children's research hospital) presented preliminary results of using bevacizumab in combination with neoadjuvant chemotherapy (two courses of IDA) in 27 children with osteosarcoma. The drug was used at a dose of 15 mg/kg. There are three introductions for neoadjuvant chemotherapy. A satisfactory toxicity profile has been established. The study NCT00667342 continues [54, 55].

Back in 1999, employees of the Memorial Sloan-Kettering Cancer Center presented the results of a study assessing the effect of ErbB2 expression (Erb-B2 receptor tyrosine kinase 2) on the nature of the histological response after neoadjuvant polychemotherapy and on the rates of OS and BSV. The study included 53 patients. ErbB2 overexpression was detected in 42% of patients in the entire study group, in 50% with metastatic variant and in 76% at the time of detection of relapse or refractory course of the disease, and also statistically significantly correlated with poor histological response ($p = 0.02$) and BSV ($p = 0.05$). The 5-year BSV in patients with a localized version of osteosarcoma and ErbB2-positive status was 47%, with ErbB2-negative status—79% [40].

Conflicting data on the prognostic significance of ErbB2-positive status in patients with localized osteosarcoma were obtained.

In 2002, the Japanese Osteosarcoma Group (Japanese Osteosarcoma Group) published the results of a study that included 155 patients with localized osteosarcoma from 1984 to 1995. At the same time, 5-year BSV in patients with ErbB2-positive status was 45%, with ErbB2-negative status—72% [56].

In 2014, the Children Oncology Group (COG) presented completely different results of the study, which from 1999 to 2002 included 135 patients with localized osteosarcoma. Only 13% of patients showed ErbB2-positive status. The 5-year RR in patients with ErbB2-positive status was 73%, and with the ErbB2-negative status—72%, the 5-year RR was 59 and 69%, respectively. No statistically significant difference in survival was observed [57].

Thus, it was confirmed that ErbB2 can be considered as a potential target for targeted therapy in metastatic variant, relapse, and refractory course of the disease.

COG presented the results of a phase 2 clinical trial of the drug Trastuzumab (Herceptin) in combination with MAPIE polychemotherapy in 96 patients with primary metastatic osteosarcoma. This study was conducted from 2001 to 2005.

Trastuzumab is a partially humanized IgG1κ monoclonal antibody to ErbB2, which also realizes its activity through a second type of immunopathological reaction (antibody-mediated complement-dependent cytotoxicity and antibody-mediated cell-dependent cytotoxicity). The drug was administered at a dose of 4 mg/kg in the first week, and then 2 mg/kg 1 time per week (34 in total) only in patients in whose tumor substrate ErbB2 expression was detected.

Surgical removal of the primary tumor lesion was performed at week 11. Adjuvant chemotherapy began at week 13.

In the group with trastuzumab, a good histological response was detected in 56% of patients and without trastuzumab, it was 40%, a poor histological response of 44–60%, respectively. At the same time, the 3-year OS and BSV in the group of patients who received treatment with trastuzumab accounted for 59 and 32%, and in the group of patients who received treatment without trastuzumab for 50 and 32%. Consequently, the use of trastuzumab with polychemotherapy MAPIE led to an increase in the frequency of achieving a good histological response, but not to an increase in the rates of OS and EFS [58].

Of particular interest is tumor-modifying therapy using nitrogen-containing bisphosphonates. Currently, the following mechanisms of action of nitrogen-containing bisphosphonates have been identified, which are represented by the activation of tumor cell apoptosis by the caspase mechanism (indirectly through protein Rb and P53) and without the participation of the caspase mechanism (an increase in AIF—apoptosis of the inducing factor); increased expression of TNF-related apoptosis-inducing ligand–death receptor 5 (TRAIL-DR5, TRAIL-induced apoptosis); reduction of receptor activator of nuclear factor kappa-B ligand (RANKL) expression–ligand of nuclear factor activation receptor kB in osteosarcoma cells, which leads to suppression of tumor cell proliferation, osteoclast activity, changes in the tumor microenvironment, bone resorption, and risk of metastasis; γδT activation of cellular cytotoxicity; and tumor activation of associated macrophages [59–62].

In addition, the potentiating effect of nitrogen-containing bisphosphonates on cisplatin and adriamycin has been confirmed [63].

Currently, a rather small experience has been gained in using these drugs in children with osteosarcoma.

Meyers et al. published the results of a study on the combined use of pamidronate with MAP chemotherapy. The study included 40 patients, 32 in the age group under 18, 29 with a localized version of osteosarcoma, and 11 with a primary metastatic option of osteosarcoma.

In accordance with the program, pamidronate was administered once a month at a dose of 2 mg/kg 48–72 h after adriamycin, methotrexate, a total of 12 administrations.

Surgical removal of the primary tumor lesion was performed at week 11. Adjuvant chemotherapy began at week 13. Removal of metastatic foci was carried out individually at the stage of adjuvant therapy.

The frequency of achieving a good and poor histological response is not indicated. However, relatively high rates of 5-year OS and EFS were obtained: 93 and 72% in patients with localized osteosarcoma and 64 and 45% in patients with metastatic osteosarcoma [26].

COG presented the results of the pilot protocol AOST06P1 aimed at studying the combined use of zoledronic acid with MAPIE polychemotherapy in children with the primary metastatic osteosarcoma. This study included 24 patients. Zoledronic acid was administered at a dose of 1.2–3.5 mg/m^2 in each course of chemotherapy.

The maximum tolerated dose of zoledronic acid was established, which was 2.3 mg/m^2. Indicators of a 2-year OV and EFS were 60 and 32%, respectively [63].

Piperno-Neumann et al. presented the results of a phase 3 randomized study OS 2006, the purpose of which was to identify the potentiating effect of zoledronic acid when used together with polychemotherapy MIE and MAP.

The study included 217 children, 107 in the control group, and 110 in the group with zoledronic acid. Groups of patients were statistically significantly comparable by sex, age, foci of primary and metastatic lesions, and histological variant of the tumor.

Zoledronic acid was administered at a dose of 0.05 mg/kg (maximum dose of 4 mg) with each course of chemotherapy (IE and AP).

Neoadjuvant chemotherapy consisted of two courses of IE (ifosfamide (I) 12 g/m^2, etoposide 300 mg/m^2) and seven administrations of high-dose methotrexate ((M) 12 g/m^2). Surgical removal of the primary tumor lesion was performed at week 14. Adjuvant chemotherapy included two courses of MIE in the group with a good histological response and five courses of MAP in the group with a poor histological response. A good histological response after neoadjuvant polychemotherapy was achieved in 73% of patients. However, there was no statistically significant difference in achieving a good histological response, in terms of OS and BSV in groups of patients who received programmed treatment with or without zoledronic acid. The number of events in the group with zoledronic acid was 42% (47/110) and in the group without zoledronic acid was 31% (34/107). Consequently, this study shows the high effectiveness of chemotherapy courses with IE in combination with methotrexate in the neoadjuvant regimen. The presence of the potentiating effect of zoledronic acid has not been proven [64].

In the treatment of refractory forms of osteosarcoma, drugs are also used that affect various cellular signaling pathways. Understanding the mechanisms of tumor activation opens up the possibility of using multikinase and mammalian target of rapamycin complex (mTOR) inhibitors.

Takagi and Peng et al. in an in vitro experiment on cell lines (SaOS2, MG63, HOS), pathogenetic mechanisms of cytokine-induced tumor transformation and proliferation were shown through the activation of VEGF/VEGFR/PI3K (phosphatidylinositol-4,5-bisphosphate 3-kinase)/AKT (protein kinase B) and the platelet-derived growth factor receptor (PDGFR)/PI3K/AKT signaling pathways [65, 66]. The most studied drugs from this group are currently sorafenib (nexavar) and everolimus (afinitor) [67]. Sorafenib is a nonselective multikinase inhibitor that inhibits the activity of various cellular signaling pathways, in particular VEGFR1, VEGFR2, PDGFRα, and PDGFRβ, while everolimus is an mTOR inhibitor [68].

Ymera et al. of the Italian Sarcoma Group published the results of a preclinical study (in vitro and in vivo), which noted the mutually potentiating antitumor effect of everolimus and sorafenib on osteosarcoma cell lines (KHOS, MNNG-HOS, and U2OS). The effect of everolimus and sorafenib on mTORC1/mTORC2 is manifested in a decrease in the expression of mTORC1 and an increase in the expression of mTORC2, which provides proapoptotic and antiproliferative effects. With the combined use of everolimus and sorafenib, there is a decrease in the expression of both mTORC1 and mTORC2 [69].

From 2008 to 2009, Grignani et al. of the Italian Sarcoma Group conducted a second phase of clinical trials of the drug sorafenib in patients with relapse and refractory osteosarcoma. The study included 35 patients with osteosarcoma in the age group over 14 years. Partial response was achieved in 5 (14%) patients and stabilization of the disease in 12 (34%) patients. The overall response rate was 48%. At the same time, 4-month progression-free survival was 45% (15 out of 35) [70].

From 2011 to 2013, Grignani et al. conducted a second phase of clinical trials of a combination of drugs of everolimus and sorafenib in patients with relapse and refractory osteosarcoma after performing standard polychemotherapy MAP (study NCT01804374). The study included 38 patients over the age of 18 years. Everolimus was administered in a dose of 5 mg once a day and sorafenib 400 mg two times a day. The duration of chemotherapy was 28 days. Partial response was achieved in 4 (10%) patients and stabilization of the disease in 20 (53%) patients. The overall response rate is 63%. This figure is 15% more than in the study, where sorafenib was used in monomode. A 4-month progression-free survival was 58% and for 6-month, it was 45% (17 out of 38) [71].

Thus, taking into account the data of studies in 2008 (application of sorafenib in mono mode) and 2011 (using a combination of sorafenib with everolimus), it can be said that the combination of sorafenib with everolimus leads to an increase in the overall response rate and an increase in survival rate without disease progression within 6 months. However, by the year, this difference disappears.

At ASCO 2016, preliminary results were presented in a pilot study of the use of everolimus/sorafenib in children with relapse and refractory osteosarcoma, which was carried out at the Institute of Pediatric Oncology and Hematology N.N. Blokhin Medical Research Center of Oncology from 2013 to 2016. This protocol included 14 patients. The first line of therapy is represented by the program "Osteosarcoma 2006" in seven patients and "Osteosarcoma 2014" in seven patients. All patients underwent therapy, which included doxorubicin, cisplatin, high-dose methotrexate, high-dose ifosfamide, and gemcitabine and docetaxel.

The number of courses of therapy for everolimus/sorafenib ranged from 2 to 18. The toxicity of therapy was erythema cutaneous in all patients (100%), palmar and plantar syndrome in 1 (7%), and mucositis 1–2 in 4 (28.5%). Hematologic toxicity did not exceed 1–2 degree in all patients. A transient increase in transaminases up to five norms in all patients (100%) was also noted.

Partial response to treatment was achieved in 5 of 14 (35.7%) patients and stabilization of the disease in 9 (64.3%). The overall response rate was 100%. Survival without disease progression for more than 6 months was detected in 6 out of 14 (43%) patients. The mean follow-up was 7 ± 1.2 months. The maximum period without progression of the disease is 18.4 months.

The findings suggest that everolimus/sorafenib combination resulted in a partial response in 35.7% of cases with a satisfactory toxicity profile [72].

Compared to international data (Italian sarcoma group) in the presented study, the achievement of a partial response, stabilization of the disease, and the overall response rate were significantly higher.

Currently, a number of studies aimed at studying the role of tumor-associated macrophages. Activation of tumor-associated macrophages can be achieved through the use of preparations of liposomal tripeptides (mifamurtide) and interferon preparations (interferon alpha-2A).

Meyers et al. presented the results of the randomized study CCG 7921/POG 9351, which was conducted from 1993 to 1997. The study included 662 patients with a localized version of osteosarcoma.

A feature of line A therapy was the use of two courses of neoadjuvant chemotherapy for MAP, and in line B therapy, two courses of neoadjuvant chemotherapy MAi, alternating courses of MAR and MAi at the stage of adjuvant chemotherapy, was used. Surgical removal of the primary tumor lesion was performed at week 10. Mifamurtide (MTP) was administered at a dose of 2 mg/m^2 two times a week for 12 weeks, and then once a week for 24 weeks in accordance with randomization.

The mechanism of action of mythamurtide (MTP) is to activate monocytes/macrophages with antitumor activity, which is realized by binding to specific receptors toll-like receptor 4 (TLR4) and nucleotide-binding oligomerization domain 2 receptor (NOD2), followed by altering the activity of cellular signal pathways (ERK1/2—extracellular-signal regulated kinase 1/2), NF-kB—nuclear factor kappa-B, and AP1—adapter protein 1 [73].

After removal of the primary tumor focus, a good histological response in group A was achieved in 42% of patients and in group B in 48%, and a poor histological response in group A was 58% and in group B was 52%. At the same time, the 6-year-old RH was 74%, without the use of MTP was 70% and with the MTP was 78%; BSV was 64%, without the use of MTR was 61% and with MTP was 67%. In group A: OS without the use of MTR was 71% and with MTR was 75%; BSV without MTR was 64% and with MTR was 63%. In group B: OS without the use of MTR was 71% and with MTR was 75%; BSV without MTR was 64% and with MTR was 63%.

Authors	Agents
Ferrari S.	Ifosfamide, adriamycin, cisplatin
Le Deley M.C.	Methotrexate, adriamycin, ifosfamide, etoposide
Cui Q.	Cisplatin
Pitano-Garcia A.	Doxorubicin, cisplatin
Wu X.	Methotrexate, cisplatin, adriamycin
Ohba T.	Bevacizumab (Avastin)
Children Oncology Group	Trastuzumab

Table 3.
Trials/authors and agents.

The addition of MTP to polychemotherapy led to a statistically significant increase in the 6-year OS from 70 to 78% ($p = 0.03$), and there was also a tendency to an increase in BSV, mainly in group B ($p = 0.08$) [25].

Kubo et al. published the results of a pilot study that determined the prognostic significance of the expression level of interferon α/β receptors in 40 patients with localized osteosarcoma who received treatment according to the NECO95J program. Expression of interferon α/β receptors was detected in 45% of patients. When conducting multivariate statistical analysis, a significant association was observed between the expression of interferon α/β receptors and 5-year-old OM and survival free of metastatic lesions (VSMP). The 5-year OM, in the presence of expression of the α/β interferon receptor in the tumor substrate, was 81%, with no expression, 47% ($p = 0.043$), and in the 5-year HSMP, it was 75 and 41% ($p = 0.023$). This study confirms the possibility of using interferon preparations in the treatment of osteosarcoma in patients with overexpression of α/β interferon receptors [74].

Bielack et al. presented the results of the EURAMOS1 study in patients with a good histological response after neoadjuvant MAP chemotherapy. In the age group up to 30 years, the MAP line of therapy was carried out to 359 patients, the MAP INF line α–2b—to 357 patients, in the age group up to 20 years—333 (92.7%) and 332 (92.9%) patients. Groups of patients are statistically significantly comparable by sex, age, localization of the primary tumor lesion, the presence of metastatic lesions, and the histological variant of the tumor.

In accordance with the program, pegylated INF–α–2b was administered at a dose of 0.5 mg/kg (at a maximum dose of 50 mg) once a week for 4 weeks, and then 1 mg/kg (at a maximum dose of 100 mg) 1 time per week (from 30 to 104 weeks of programmed treatment).

In a group of 630 patients with a localized version of osteosarcoma, 135 events were detected: 72 in patients who received the MAP therapy line and 63 in patients who received the MAP INF therapy line–2b. At the same time, the 3-year EFS was 77 and 80%, respectively. Therefore, the use of INF–α–2b as maintenance therapy after MAP in patients with a good histological response did not lead to an increase in EFS [75].

The data set out in paragraph 3 are summarized in **Table 3**.

4. Conclusion

Thus, the results of treatment of children with primary metastatic osteosarcoma, relapse, and refractory course of the disease remain unsatisfactory. Molecular biological factors that determine sensitivity to chemotherapy, invasive, and metastatic potential of the tumor, as well as the prognosis of the disease, among which special attention is deserved are as follows: expression of MGMT protein, methylation of the promoter part of the MGMT gene, expression of ERCC1 proteins, VEGF, CD133, p-STAT3tyr705, C-MYC, expression of RFC1 micro-RNA, and the presence of rearrangement of the TOR2A gene. It is important to note that there was no comprehensive assessment of the value of these markers for the histological response to neoadjuvant chemotherapy and survival rates in patients with osteosarcoma.

Author details

Maxim Yu. Rykov[1,2]* and Elmira R. Sengapova[1]

1 Institute of Pediatric Oncology and Hematology, N.N. Blokhin Medical Research Center of Oncology, Moscow, Russian Federation

2 I.M. Sechenov First Moscow State Medical University (Sechenov University), Moscow, Russian Federation

*Address all correspondence to: wordex2006@rambler.ru

References

[1] Isakoff MS, Bielack SS, Meltzer P, et al. Osteosarcoma: Current treatment and a collaborative pathway to success. Journal of Clinical Oncology. 2015;**33**(27):3029-3035. DOI: 10.1200/JCO.2014.59.4895

[2] Punanov YA, Andreeva TV, Gafton GI, et al. The results of combined therapy in children and adolescents with osteosarcoma. Oncopediatrics. 2014;**1**(2):49-53. (In Russian)

[3] Doyle LA. Sarcoma classification: An update based on the 2013 World Health Organization classification of tumors of soft tissue and bone. Cancer. 2014;**120**(12):1763-1774. DOI: 10.1002/cncr.28657

[4] Fletcher CDM, Bridge JA, Hogendoorn JA, et al. Pathology and Genetics of Tumours of Soft Tissue and Bone. WHO Classification 2013. Available from: http://apps.who.int/bookorders/anglais/detart1.jsp?codlan=1&codcol=70&codcch=4005

[5] Ritter J, Bielack SS, et al. Osteosarcoma. Annals of Oncology. 2010;**21**:320-325. DOI: 10.1093/annonc/mdq276

[6] Fletcher CDM et al. Pathology and Genetics of Tumours of Soft Tissue and Bone. WHO Classification 2013. Available from: http:/sarcomahclp.org/reviews/who-classification-sarcomas.html

[7] Gress DM, Edge SB, Gershenwald JE, et al. Principles of cancer staging. In: Amin MB, Edge SB, Greene FL, et al., editors. AJCC Cancer Staging Manual. 8th ed. New York: Springer; 2017. pp. 3-30

[8] Avella M, Bacci G, McDonald DJ, et al. Adjuvant chemotherapy with six drugs (Adriamycin, methotrexate, cisplatinum, bleomycin, cyclophosphamide and dactinomycin) for non-metastatic high grade osteosarcoma of the extremities. Results of 32 patients and comparison to 127 patients concomitantly treated with the same drugs in a neoadjuvant form. Chemioterapia. 1988;**7**(2):133-137

[9] Fuchs N, Bielack SS, Epler D, et al. Long-term results of the co-operative German-Austrian-Swiss osteosarcoma study group's protocol COSS-86 of intensive multidrug chemotherapy and surgery for osteosarcoma of the limbs. Annals of Oncology. 1998;**9**:893-899

[10] Ngan RKC. Chemotherapy for non-metastatic high-grade osteosarcoma of extremity—Is neoadjuvant better than adjuvant? Hong Kong Journal of Radiology. 2003;**6**:7-14

[11] Pratt CB, Meyer WH, Rao BN, et al. Osteosarcoma studies at St. Jude Children's research hospital from 1968 through 1990. Cancer Treatment and Research. 1993;**62**:323-326

[12] Saeter G, Alvegard TA, Elomaa I, et al. Treatment of osteosarcoma of the extremities with the T-10 protocol, with emphasis on the effect of preoperative chemotherapy with single-agent high-dose methotrexate: A Scandinavian Sarcoma Group Study. Journal of Clinical Oncology. 1991;**9**(10):1766-1775. DOI: 10.1200/JCO.1991.9.10.1766

[13] Souhami RL, Craft AW, der Eijken JWV, et al. Randomised trial of two regimens of chemotherapy inoperable osteosarcoma: A study of the European Osteosarcoma Intergroup. The Lancet. 1997;**350**:911-917. DOI: 10.1016/S0140-6736(97)02307-6

[14] Bacci G, Ferrari S, Bertoni F, et al. Long-term outcome for patients with nonmetastatic osteosarcoma of the extremity treated at the Istituto Ortopedico Rizzoli according to

the Istituto Ortopedico Rizzoli/Osteosarcoma-2 protocol: An updated report. Journal of Clinical Oncology. 2000;**18**(24):4016-4027. DOI: 10.1200/JCO.2000.18.24.4016

[15] Ferrari S, Ruqqieri P, Cefalo G, et al. Neoadjuvant chemotherapy with methotrexate, cisplatin, and doxorubicin with or without Ifosfamide in nonmetastatic osteosarcoma of the extremity: An Italian Sarcoma Group Trial ISG/OS-1. Journal of Clinical Oncology. 2012;**30**(17):2112-2118. DOI: 10.1200/JCO.2011.38.4420

[16] Ferrari S, Smeland S, Mercuri M, et al. Neoadjuvant chemotherapy with high-dose Ifosfamide, high-dose methotrexate, cisplatin, and doxorubicin for patients with localized osteosarcoma of the extremity: A joint study by the Italian and Scandinavian Sarcoma Groups. Journal of Clinical Oncology. 2005;**23**(34):8845-8852. DOI: 10.1200/JCO.2004.00.5785

[17] Hegyi M, Semsei AF, Jakab Z, et al. Good prognosis of localized osteosarcoma in young patients treated with limb-salvage surgery and chemotherapy. Pediatric Blood & Cancer. 2011;**57**:415-422. DOI: 10.1002/pbc.23172

[18] Smeland S, Bruland OS, Hjorth L, et al. Results of the Scandinavian Sarcoma Group XIV protocol for classical osteosarcoma. Acta Orthopaedica. 2011;**82**(2):211-216. DOI: 10.3109/17453674.2011.566141

[19] Iwamoto Y, Tanaka K, Isu K, et al. Multiinstitutional phase II study of neoadjuvant chemotherapy for osteosarcoma (NECO study) in Japan: NECO-93J and NECO-95J. Journal of Orthopedic Science. 2009;**14**:397-404. DOI: 10.1007/s00776-009-1347-6

[20] Petrilli S, de Camargo B, Filho VO, et al. Results of the Brazilian osteosarcoma treatment group studies III and IV: Prognostic factors and impact on survival. Journal of Clinical Oncology. 2006;**24**(7):1161-1168. DOI: 10.1200/JCO.2005.03.5352

[21] Goorin AM, Shwartzentruber DJ, Devidas M, et al. Presurgical chemotherapy compared with immediate surgery and adjuvant chemotherapy for nonmetastatic osteosarcoma: Pediatric Oncology Group Study POG-8651. Journal of Clinical Oncology. 2003;**21**:1574-1580. DOI: 10.1200/JCO.2003.08.165

[22] Le Deley MC, Guinebretiere JM, Gentet VC, et al. SFOP OS94: A randomised trial comparing preoperative high-dose methotrexate plus doxorubicin to high-dose methotrexate plus etoposide and ifosfamide in osteosarcoma patients. European Journal of Cancer. 2007;**43**:752-761. DOI: 10.1016/j.ejca.2006.10.023

[23] Hinds PS, Gattuso JS, Billups CA, et al. Aggressive treatment of non-metastatic osteosarcoma improves health-related quality of life in children and adolescents. European Journal of Cancer. 2009;**45**:2007-2014. DOI: 10.1016/j.ejca.2009.04.020

[24] Daw NC, Neel MD, Rao BN, et al. Frontline treatment of localized osteosarcoma without methotrexate: Results of the St. Jude Children's Research Hospital OS99 trial. Cancer. 2011;**117**(12):2770-2778. DOI: 10.1002/cncr.25715

[25] Meyers PA, Schwartz CL, Krailo MD, et al. Osteosarcoma: The addition of muramyl tripeptide to chemotherapy improves overall survival—A report from the Children's Oncology Group. Journal of Clinical Oncology. 2008;**28**(9):633-638. DOI: 10.1200/JCO.2008.14.0095

[26] Meyers PA, Healeya JH, Choua AJ, et al. Addition of pamidronate to

chemotherapy for the treatment of osteosarcoma. Cancer. 2011;**117**(8):1736-1744. DOI: 10.1002/cncr.25744

[27] Isakoff MS, Barkauskas DA, Ebb D, et al. Poor survival for osteosarcoma of the pelvis: A report from the Children's Oncology Group. Clinical Orthopedics Related Research. 2012;**470**:2007-2013. DOI: 10.1007/s11999-012-2284-9

[28] Boye K, Del Prever AB, Eiksson E, et al. High-dose chemotherapy with stem cell rescue in the primary treatment of metastatic and pelvic osteosarcoma: Final results of the ISG/SSG II Study. Pediatric Blood & Cancer. 2014;**61**(5):840-845. DOI: 10.1002/pbc.24868

[29] Smeland S, Whelan JS, Bielack SS, et al. Event-free survival and overall survival in 2,253 patients with osteosarcoma registered to EURAMOS-1. Journal of Clinical Oncology. 2015;**33**(suppl):abstr 10512. http://meetinglibrary.asco.org/content/143782-156

[30] Whelan JS, Bielack SS, Marina N, et al. EURAMOS-1, an International Randomised Study for osteosarcoma: Results from pre-randomisation treatment. Annals of Oncology. 2015;**26**:407-414. DOI: 10.1093/annonc/mdu526

[31] Ferrari S, Meazza C, Palmerini E, et al. Nonmetastatic osteosarcoma of the extremity. Neoadjuvant chemotherapy with methotrexate, cisplatin, doxorubicin and ifosfamide. An Italian Sarcoma Group (ISG/OS-oss). Tumori. 2014;**100**:612-618. DOI: 10.1700/1778.19262

[32] Goorin AM, Harris MB, Bernstein M, et al. Phase II/III trial of etoposide and high-dose ifosfamide in newly diagnosed metastatic osteosarcoma: A pediatric oncology group trial. Journal of Clinical Oncology. 2002;**2**:426-433. DOI: 10.1200/JCO.2002.20.2.426

[33] Marina NM, Smeland S, Bielack SS, et al. Comparison of MAPIE versus MAP in patients with poor response to preoperative chemotherapy for newly diagnosed high-grade osteosarcoma (EURAMOS1): An open-label, International, Randomized Controlled Trial. Lancet Oncology. 2016;**17**(10):1396-1408. DOI: 10.1016/S1470-2045(16)30214-5

[34] Cui Q, Jiang W, Guo J, et al. Relationship between hypermetylated MGMT gene and osteosarcoma necrosis rate after chemotherapy. Pathology and Oncology Research. 2011;**17**:587-591. DOI: 10.1007/s12253-010-9354-7

[35] Cui Q, Li D, Liu C, et al. The significance of MGMT protein detection in evaluation of osteosarcoma necrosis rate after cisplatin chemotherapy. Bosnian Journal of Basic Medical Sciences. 2011;**11**(2):80-83

[36] Hattinger CM, Michelacci F, Sella F, et al. ERCC1 protein expression predicts survival in patients with high-grade, non-metastatic osteosarcoma treated with neoadjuvant chemotherapy. Histopathology. 2015;**67**(3):338-347. DOI: 10.1111/his.12653

[37] Nguyen A, Lasthaus C, Guerin E, et al. Role of topoisomerases in pediatric high grade osteosarcomas: TOP2A gene is one of the unique molecular biomarkers of chemoresponse. Cancer. 2013;**5**:662-675. DOI: 10.3390/cancers5020662

[38] Pitano-Garcia A, Zalacain M, Marrodan L, et al. Methotrexate in pediatric osteosarcoma: Response and toxicity in relation to genetic polymorphisms and dihydrofolate reductase and reduced folate carrier 1 expression. Journal of Pediatrics. 2009;**154**(5):688-693. DOI: 10.1016/j.jpeds.2008

[39] Xiao X, Wang W, Zhang H, et al. Individualized chemotherapy for

osteosarcoma and identification of gene mutations in osteosarcoma. Tumour Biology. 2015;**36**(4):2437-2435. DOI: 10.1007/s13277-014-2853-5

[40] Gorlick R, Huvos AG, Heller G, et al. Expression of HER2/erbB-2 correlates with survival in osteosarcoma. Journal of Clinical Oncology. 1999;**17**:2781-2788. DOI: 10.1200/JCO.1999.17.9.2781

[41] He A, Qi W, Huang Y, et al. CD133 expression predicts lung metastases and poor prognosis in osteosarcoma patients: A clinical and experimental study. Experimental and Therapeutic Medicine. 2012;**4**:435-441. DOI: 10.3892/etm.2012.603

[42] Rossi B, Schinzari G, Maccauro G, et al. Neoadjuvant multidrug chemotherapy including high-dose methotrexate modifies VEGF expression in osteosarcoma: An immunihistochemical analysis. BMC Musculoskeletal Disorders. 2010;**11**:34. https://www.ncbi. nlm.nih. gov/pmc/articles/PMC2835659/pdf/1471-2474-11-34.pdf

[43] Tu B, Du L, Fan QM, et al. STAT3 activation by IL6 from mesenchymal stem cell promotes the proliferation and metastasis of osteosarcoma. Cancer Letters. 2012;**325**:80-88. DOI: 10.1016/j. canlet.2012.06.006

[44] Yang R, Qin J, Hoang BH, et al. Polymorphism and methylation of the reduced folate carrier in osteosarcoma. Clinical Orthopedics Related Research. 2008;**466**:2046-2051. DOI: 10.1007/s11999-008-0323-3

[45] Abarategi A, Tornin J, Martinez-Cruzado L, et al. Osteosarcoma: Cells of origin, cancer stem cells, and target therapies. Stem Cells International. 2016;**2016**:1-13. https://www.hindawi. com/journals/sci/2016/3631764

[46] Fan H, Liu G, Zhao C, et al. Transcription factor OCT4 promotes osteosarcoma by regulating IncRNAAK055347. Oncology Letters. 2017;**13**:396-402. DOI: 10.3892/ol.2016.5400

[47] PosthumaDeBoer J, van Royen BJ, Helder MN, et al. Mechanisms of therapy resistance in osteosarcoma: A review. Oncology Discovery. 2013;**1**:8. http://www.hoajonline.com/journals/pdf/2052-6199-1-8.pdf

[48] Li JI, Zhong XY, Li ZY, et al. CD133 expression in osteosarcoma and derivation of CD133 cells. Molecular Medicine Reports. 2013;**7**:577-584. DOI: 10.3892/mmr.2012.1231

[49] Tu B, Zhu J, Liu S, et al. Mesenchymal stem cells promote osteosarcoma cell survival and drug resistance through activation of STAT3. Oncotarget. 2016;**7**(30):48296-48308. DOI: 10.18632/oncotarget.10219

[50] Han G, Wang Y, Bi W, et al. C-MYC overexpression promotes osteosarcoma cell invasion via activation of MEK-ERK pathway. Oncology Research. 2012;**20**:149-156. DOI: 10.3727/096504012X13522227232237

[51] Wu X, Cai ZD, Lou LM, et al. Expressions of p53, C-MYC, BCL2 and apoptotic index in human osteosarcoma and their correlations with prognosis of patients. Cancer Epidemiology. 2012;**36**:212-216. DOI: 10.1016/j. canep.2011.08.002

[52] Ohba T, Cates AMM, Cole HA, et al. Autocrine VEGF/VEGFR1 signaling in a subpopulation of cell associates with aggressive osteosarcoma. Molecular Cancer Research. 2014;**12**(8):1100-1111. DOI: 10.1158/1541-7786.MCR-14-0037

[53] Han K, Peyret T, Quartino A, et al. Bevacizumab dosing strategy in pediatric cancer patients based on population pharmacokinetic analysis with external validation. British Journal of Clinical Pharmacology.

2015;**81**:148-160. DOI: 10.1111/bcp.12778

[54] Bishop M. A Study of Bevacizumab in Combination with Chemotherapy for Treatment of Osteosarcoma. Available from: https://clinicaltrials.gov/ct2/show/study/NCT00667342

[55] Akatsuka T, Wada T, Kokai Y, et al. ErbB2 expression is correlated with increased survival of patients with osteosarcoma. Cancer. 2002;**94**:1397-1404. DOI: 10.1002/cncr.10360

[56] Turner DC, Navid F, Daw NC, et al. Population pharmacokinetics of bevacizumab in children with osteosarcoma: Implications for dosing. Clinical Cancer Research. 2014;**20**(10):2783-27924. DOI: 10.1158/1078-0432

[57] Gorlick S, Barkauskas DA, Krailo M, et al. HER-2 expression is not prognostic in osteosarcoma; a Children's Oncology Group Prospective Biology Study. Pediatric Blood & Cancer. 2014;**61**:1558-1564. DOI: 10.1002/pbc.25074

[58] Ebb D, Holcombe G, Karen M, et al. Phase II trial of trastuzumab in combination with cytotoxic chemotherapy for treatment of metastatic osteosarcoma with human epidermal growth factor receptor 2 overexpression: A report from the Children's Oncology Group. Journal of Clinical Oncology. 2012;**30**(20):2245 2551. DOI: 10.1200/JCO.2011.37.4546

[59] Akiyama T, Dass CR, Choong PF, et al. Novel therapeutic strategy for osteosarcoma targeting osteoclast differentiation, bone-resorbing activity, and apoptosis pathway. Molecular Cancer Therapy. 2008;**7**(11):3461-3469. DOI: 10.1158/1535-7163.MCT-08-0530

[60] Clezardin P, Benzaid I, Croucher PI, et al. Bisphosphonates in preclinical bone oncology. Bone. 2011;**49**:66-70. DOI: 10.1016/j.bone.2010.11.017

[61] Lee JA, Jung JS, Kim DH, et al. RANKL expression is related to treatment outcome of patients with localized, high-grade osteosarcoma. Pediatric Blood & Cancer. 2010;**56**:738-743. DOI: 10.1002/pbc.22720

[62] Li Z et al. Potential of human γδ T cells for immunotherapy of osteosarcoma. Molecular Biology Reports. 2013;**40**:427-437. DOI: 10.1007/s11033-012-2077-y

[63] Goldsby RE, Fan TM, Vallaluna D, et al. Feasibility and dose discovery analysis of zoledronic acid with concurrent hemotherapy in the treatment of newly diagnosed metastatic osteosarcoma: A report from the Children's Oncology Group. European Journal of Cancer. 2013;**49**:2384-2391. DOI: 10.1016/j.ejca.2013.03.018

[64] Piperno-Neumann S, Le Deley MC, Redini F, et al. Zoledronate in combination with chemotherapy and surgery to treat osteosarcoma (OS2006): A randomized, multicenter, open-label, phase 3 trial. Lancet Oncology. 2016;**17**(8):1070-1080. DOI: 10.1016/S1470-2045(16)30096-1

[65] Peng N, Gao S, Guo X, et al. Silencing of VEGF inhibits human osteosarcoma angiogenesis and promotes cell apoptosis via VEGF/PI3K/AKT signaling pathway. American Journal of Translational Research. 2016;**8**(2):1005-1015

[66] Takagi S, Ai T, Takami M, et al. Platelets promote osteosarcoma cell growth through activation of the platelet-derived growth factor receptor-AKT signaling axis. Cancer Science. 2014;**105**(8):983-988. DOI: 10.1111/cas.12464

[67] Shaikh AB, Li F, Li M, et al. Present advances and future perspectives of molecular target therapy for osteosarcoma. International Journal of

Molecular Sciences. 2016;**17**(4):1-21. https://www.ncbi.nlm.nih.gov/pubmed/2705853

[68] Kansara M, Teng MW, Smith MJ, et al. Translational biology of osteosarcoma. Nature Reviews Cancer. 2014;**14**:722-735. DOI: 10.1038/nrc3838

[69] Ymera P, Dell'Aglio C, Basirico M, et al. The combination of sorafenib and everolimus abrogates mTORC1 and mTORC2 upregulation in osteosarcoma preclinical models. Clinical Cancer Research. 2013;**19**(8):2117-2131. DOI: 10.1158/1078-0432

[70] Grignani G, Palmerini E, Dileo P, et al. A phase II trial of sorafenib in relapsed and unresectable high-grade osteosarcoma after failure of standard multimodal therapy: An Italian Sarcoma Group Study. Annals of Oncology. 2012;**23**(2):508-516. DOI: 10.1093/annonc/mdr151

[71] Grignani G, Palmerini E, Ferraresi V, et al. Sorafenib and everolimus for patients with unresectable high-grade osteosarcoma progressing after standard treatment: A non-randomised phase 2 clinical trial. Lancet Oncology. 2015;**16**:98-107. DOI: 10.1016/S1470-2045(14)71136-2

[72] Fedenko A et al. Everolimus/sorafenib combination in the treatment of pediatric osteosarcomas: Singke center experience. Journal of Clinical Oncology. 2016;**34**(suppl):abstr e22501. http://meetinglibrary.asco.org/content/167657-176

[73] Ando K, Mori K, Corradini N, et al. Mifamurtide for the treatment of nonmetastatic osteosarcoma. Expert Opinion on Pharmacotherapy. 2011;**12**:285-292. DOI: 10.1517/14656566.2011.543129

[74] Kubo T, Shimose S, Matsuo T, et al. Interferon–α/β receptor as a prognostic marker in osteosarcoma. The Journal of Bone and Joint Surgery. American Volume. 2011;**93**:519-526. DOI: 10.2106/JBJS.J.00198

[75] Bielack SS, Smeland S, Whelan JS, et al. Methotrexate, doxorubicin and cisplatin (MAP) plus maintenance pegylated interferon α–2b versus MAP alone in patients with resectable high-grade osteosarcoma and good histologic response to preoperative MAP: First results of the EURAMOS1 good response randomized controlled trial. Journal of Clinical Oncology. 2015;**33**(20):2279-2287. DOI: 10.1200/JCO.2014.60.0734